5-HTP
The Serotonin Connection

*The Exciting New Approach to
Overcoming Depression, Reducing Anxiety,
Controlling Your Appetite, Sleep Disorders,
Hostility & Aggression, Addictions,
Memory Loss , Headaches,
Fibromyalgia & Chronic Fatigue Syndrome,
Premenstrual Syndrome and Menopause.*

OTHNIEL J. SEIDEN, M.D. &
Jane L. Bilett, PhD, Clinical Psychologist

Copyright 2013
Othniel J. Seiden, MD & Jane L. Bilett, Ph.D.

All rights reserved

ISBN: 1519148445

FOREWORD

Alternative medicine, its methods, and its medicinals are all too often sensationalized. Extremists, health food purveyors, promoters of herbals and supplements, manufacturers of various devices, and other zealots tend to hail every new development, discovery, or rediscovery as a panacea that will transform people's lives. On the other hand, a staunch group of overly conservative physicians are convinced that any remedy not grounded in age-old medical tradition or developed in university or hospital research lab is nothing short of charlatanism. Both opinions are equally flawed.

These latter physicians seem to have forgotten, or perhaps never learned, that many of the drugs prescribed today are manufactured chemical reproductions of remedies found in nature, which have often been used successfully by healers and physicians for many generations.

The safest ground is the middle ground. The intelligent physician, and the intelligent patient must each consider the facts and make an educated decision about new products and techniques. Recall that a few years ago the effectiveness of acupuncture was pooh-poohed by most Western physicians, who didn't think the subject worthy of consideration. Nevertheless, any procedure that has been practiced for over 4,000 years must be evaluated with an open and Impartial mind. Now that acupuncture has been scientifically tested in the West, most physicians are respectful of the technique. This is not to say that acupuncture will cure anything and everything. It is not a panacea. We have yet to find a panacea. Panaceas are few and far between. Yet acupuncture has its place in the practice of medicine, within certain limitations, and it can be very beneficial *within* those limitations.

The same is true of *5-hydroxy-tryptophan* or 5-HTP, as it is popularly known and its precursor, the *neurotransmitter Serotonin*. In recent years much has been written about 5-HTP, Serotonin, and other similar chemicals, and even more has been rumored by gossip, which is often the first wave of cutting-edge information. However all too often such information becomes sensationalized. Wish becomes supposition, suppositions became theories, and theories become facts all spread through whispers and unfounded statements. That is how "panaceas" are born. And when someone figures out how to get rich from a certain panacea, there is no stopping the frenzy.

It is not our purpose to sensationalize 5-HTP, Serotonin, or any other product. We merely intend to examine these chemicals, products, and end product, and the claims being made in connection with them, in order to provide objective data that will help you make educated decisions to live by.

CONTENTS

TRYPTOPHAN, 5-HTP, AND SEROTONIN

What is this 5-HTP phenomenon that is hardly known here in the United States? What is its relationship to tryptophan and the neurotransmitter Serotonin, which mediates and controls so many of our moods and bodily functions: appetite, anxiety, depression, sleep, and pain, to name just a few? Why has our pharmaceutical industry tended to ignore this supplement while the FDA labeled it an experimental orphan drug? Why are so many progressive physicians and researchers taking an interest in 5-HTP, the amino acid tryptophan, and Serotonin? What is behind all of the amazing claims for 5-HTP? Is it just sensationalism, or do the results justify these claims? Above all, is 5-HTP a safe product to use? These are merely a few of the questions this book will try to answer.

Why are so many progressive physicians and private researchers taking an interest in 5-HTP, the amino acid tryptophan, and serotonin?

But before we get to the meat of the matter, please bear with us while we briefly indulge in some basic chemistry, to make certain that all our readers are all of one mind. If your background in chemistry is more sophisticated than our next few paragraphs, feel free to skip ahead; otherwise, you may find the review helpful. The medicinals mentioned in this book, including 5-hydroxy-tryptophan and Serotonin are, of course, chemical compounds. Let's review a few fundamentals of chemistry so that all readers will be equipped to understand this text.

Chemistry is the science of matter, the study of the basic *elements* and the *compounds* they make up. *Inorganic chemistry* is the study of non-living matter, while *organic chemistry* studies living or previously living matter. *Biochemistry* is the study of chemical changes that occur in living or recently living matter as a function of life and death processes. *Cellular chemistry* is the science of chemical changes and events at the cellular or sub-cellular levels.

Elements are the most basic components of matter. All matter is made up of *atoms* of the various chemical elements, their *mixtures*, or their molecular *compounds*. Examples of matter that are composed of a single element are gold; silver; platinum; pure carbon in the form of coal, diamonds, or charcoal; oxygen; and hydrogen. One example of matter that is composed of mixtures of elemental atoms is air, which contains oxygen, nitrogen, hydrogen, helium, and several other gases that are mixed together; however, its atoms are not compounded together to form molecules or another substance. It is like having a mixture of sand and water. No matter how much you shake it, stir it, or cook it, you still have only sand and water mixed together; and if you filter the solution, you will get sand on one side of the filter and plain water on the other. In spite of everything you do to it, no chemical reaction occurs between the parts of the mixture that will create a new form of matter.

In chemical compounds, on the other hand, the atoms of various elements react chemically to form molecules of a new form of matter. For example, if you put together one atom of the element oxygen with two atoms of hydrogen, under the proper conditions, you create a new substance called H^2O, meaning that it has two atoms of hydrogen for each atom of oxygen. This new substance is what we know as water. Put it through a filter and what comes out the other side is still water; the filter will not separate the hydrogen and oxygen as it did the mixture of sand and water.

So much for inorganic chemistry; now that we've passed the basic course, our interests will lie mainly with organic, bio, and cellular chemistries. As was mentioned earlier, organic chemistry is the study of living or once living matter. One chemical ingredient that all living matter has in common is carbon. Whatever other elements may be compounded in molecules of living or dead matter, carbon is present. Organic com pounds make up all insects, animals, vegetables, plants, trees, cellular creatures, fungus, in fact, all that lives today and all that lived in the past. Included among organic compounds are the things we eat: the proteins, the fats, the carbohydrates, and the sugars. Our vitamins are organic; however, the minerals that we need in small or trace amounts are inorganic. Our main concern at present will be with the organic compounds known as *proteins*.

Serotonin deficiency is linked to many pathological processes; therefore, people suffering from a serotonin deficiency, or a too-rapid uptake of Serotonin can probably benefit from 5-HTP therapy. This is the theory behind most of the claims for the benefits of 5-HTP supplementation.

Proteins are contained in the meats we eat, many of the vegetables and dairy products we ingest, and some of the medicinal remedies that we rely on. Proteins are made up of *amino acids*. There are actually hundreds of amino acids, but, for the most part, we are interested in only about 20 of them. A protein that contains all 20 of these amino acids is known as a *complete protein*. Complete proteins are primarily meat and dairy proteins or proteins that have their origin in animal sources. Any protein that has less than all 20 amino acids is an incomplete protein and usually originates from a vegetable source. This does not mean that vegetarians cannot get complete proteins in their diet, because combinations of incomplete proteins can indeed provide complete protein; For example, the staple diet of many Third World countries, beans combined with rice, provides a complete protein meal.

Amino acids are also divided up into essential and nonessential amino acids. Nonessential amino acids are the ones our bodies can synthesize if they are ingested in insufficient quantities; conversely, essential amino acids are those we need for proper functioning yet cannot synthesize,, thus we must obtain them in our diet.

But why are we so concerned with amino acids? Because amino acids are the building blocks from which our bodies produce 5-HTP, the subject of this book. The tryptophan in 5-hydroxy tryptophan is one of the essential amino acids we can only acquire through our diet, whether from protein foods or from 5-HTP supplements.

The amazing part of the story is how 5-HTP then performs in the body. And that is where biochemistry and cellular chemistry come into the picture. The biochemical or chemical functions of 5-HTP occur at the *intracellular* and *intercellular* levels in our bodies. Thus, we are mostly concerned with cellular chemistry and physiology, or cellular pathology in the case of illnesses.

This ends our crash course in inorganic, organic, bio, and cellular chemistry; hopefully, everyone will have at least a basic understanding of the chemical vocabulary we may occasionally use. Since we now speak the same language, let's move on.

What Is 5-HTP?

The nickname 5-HTP stands for 5-hydroxy-tryptophan, taking the H from hydroxy, the T from trypto, and the P from phan. As was mentioned earlier, our bodies manufacture 5-HTP from the amino acids we get from proteins in our diet. The 5-HTP is a *precursor* to *Serotonin*, also called 5-HT (note that the P is gone), an important *neurotransmitter* that mediates many of our bodily functions.

So, to quickly review: (1) 5-HTP, or 5-hydroxy-tryptophan, is a breakdown product of tryptophan, an essential amino acid present in most protein foods. (2) It is a precursor to Serotonin, 5-HT. Serotonin is an important neurotransmitter that mediates many of our bodily functions.

Serotonin deficiency is linked to many pathological processes; therefore, people suffering from a Serotonin deficiency, or a too-rapid uptake of Serotonin can probably benefit from 5-HTP therapies. This is the theory behind most of the claims for the benefits of 5-HTP supplementation.

Let's take a step back and discuss just exactly what a Neurotransmitter does. Most of our bodily functions are triggered by nerve impulses from one area telling another area to do something. For example, we see someone on TV eat an apple and our eyes send impulses via the optic nerve to the brain, showing the brain the apple consumption. Our brain thinks, "That's a great idea," and so then tells us to go to the refrigerator to eat an apple. To accomplish this, the brain orders our muscles to move us to the fridge, take out the apple, and bite! Mmmm! It was a great idea!

Since 5-HTP is not even in the PDR, quite frankly, many doctors are nei ther aware of, nor very conversant with, the product. On the other hand, some physicians are using 5-HTP for Parkinson's disease, myelomas, anxiety, depression, appetite control, Alzheimer's disease, sleep disorders, autism, addictions, aggression, aging problems, dementia, and numerous other health problems.

Now at each step along the way messages were sent all over the body via the nerves, to and from the brain, to and from the eyes, to and from various muscles-literally millions of messages just to get that apple into the mouth, not to mention chewing it up, swallowing it, and, yes, even digesting it. And every nerve impulse had to be transmitted across junctions between the nerve endings and the organs or the muscles those nerve impulses stimulated. Enter our hero, serotonin!

When a nerve impulse has to cross one of these billions and trillions of junctions in our body, the nerve ending secretes a small amount of a neurotransmitter, one of which is Serotonin; this facilitates the connection and lets the impulse stimulate the end organ into action. Thus, theoretically, if there is an insufficient amount of the neurotransmitter, the end organ will not be sufficiently stimulated and will not function properly. No apple reward! Actually, the process could have failed anywhere along the line. The vision of the apple might not have stimulated your appetite. If it had stimulated your appetite, it might not have provided enough energy to get your body off the couch to go to the refrigerator. If you did get to the refrigerator, and even managed to bite, chew, and swallow the apple, perhaps there was a lack of the neurotransmitter in your intestinal tract, resulting in indigestion. Now we begin to see how many ways the neurotransmitter Serotonin can affect our well being.

There is another factor to consider, *neurotransmitter Reuptake.* Once the impulse has passed on to the end organ that is waiting to be stimulated, the cells around the junction reabsorb the neurotransmitter. This prevents overstimulation and lets the end organ be stimulated very precisely, with a fresh supply of neurotransmitter for each impulse. We will see the importance of this reuptake system later.

If a Serotonin deficiency occurs at a juncture that Serotonins mediates, then in theory the bodily function in that area will be imbalanced, and theoretically, if insufficient Serotonin causes that pathological condition or behavior, for all behavior is also mediated by neurotransmitters, then restoration of the proper quantity of neurotransmitter will restore normal physiological function, activity, and behavior. Yet nothing in the living animal is ever this simple. In some cases the defect may not be in the neurotransmitter but, rather, in a malfunction of the end organ or the organ sending the stimulation. Thankfully, in this text we will only concern ourselves with neurotransmitter problems.

Unlike tryptophan, 5-HTP is not fermented or manufactured through chemical synthesis. It is a natural extract from the seeds of the Grifonia plant.

The FDA has classified 5-HTP as an orphan drug. None of the pharmaceutical houses have a patent on 5-HTP, which probably lessens their incentive to spend much time and money researching the supplement. Since 5-HTP is not even in the PDR, quite frankly, many doctors are neither aware of, nor very conversant with, the product. On the other hand, some physicians are using 5-HTP for Parkinson's disease, myoclonus, anxiety, depression, appetite control, Alzheimer's disease, sleep disorders, autism, addictions, aggression, aging problems, dementia, and numerous other health problems. Most of this medical use of 5- HTP is considered experimental, and the number of authentic, placebo-controlled, double-blind studies of 5-HTP is limited, _ partly due to lack of funding and partly because, without patent protection, manufacturers hesitate to invest in research and development. In spite of this, it is classed as an investigational new drug (IND), so doctors who want to obtain 5-HTP and dispense it as part of a clinical investigation should get information from the Food and Drug Administration by contacting and applying for a TND# from the FDA Center for Drug Evaluation and Research, (301) 594-5460. The FDA may even supply 5-HTP free to a physician for experimental use.

To date, 5-HTP appears to have few side effects and has not shown any remarkable untoward effects in the body.

Let's look a little closer at Serotonin, specifically.

Serotonin was first isolated from the *serum* portion of blood, but it has since been found in many other cells, including in neurons, where its function most interests us. Serotonin has the property of constricting or contracting smooth muscle tissue; thus, it might be a basic factor in causing high blood pressure. Even more interesting is Serotonin's action on neuronal excitability, for this is probably how it affects behavior, mood, aggression, addiction, appetite control, and so many more of our traits, activities, and functions. Though only 1% to 2% of all the serotonin in our bodies is found in the brain, it plays an important role in mediating our behavior and moods. Serotonin is concentrated near the midline of the upper brain stem, as shown by formaldehyde-induced fluorescence, which is a microscopic histochemical study technique. It is also present in the frontal part of the brain, which is the seat of our personality. Furthermore, it affects an area of the brain called the hippocampus, where our appetite control appears to reside.

Serotonin cannot cross the blood brain barrier, which means that it cannot leave the bloodstream and pass into the brain tissue, as oxygen and other nutrients do. Therefore, the biosynthesis of brain Serotonin necessarily begins in the brain itself. For this reason, it is all the more important to ingest enough tryptophan, or 5-HTP, because the brain cannot take Serotonin from other parts of the body that may have sufficient or excess amounts of the neurotransmitter.

The first step in this biosynthesis, then, must be the dietary consumption of the amino acid tryptophan. Tryptophan, which *does* cross the blood brain barrier, is actively transported into the brain where it is hydroxylated by the action of tryptophan hydroxylase at the 5 position, yielding the isolated intermediate 5-hydroxy-tryptophan (5-HTP). Then the 5-HTP is rapidly decarboxylated by an amino acid decarboxylase to yield Serotonin, or5-HT. How all that just happened is not too important to most of us, suffice it to say, our bodies are indeed fantastic chemical laboratories!

It seems that the synthesis of 5-HTP from tryptophan is only dependent on two things: (1) the initial concentration of tryptophan and the required tryptophan hydroxylase cofactors, that is, the other chemical ingredients that are necessary to make the reaction happen; and (2) the request for 5-HTP by the brain to make sufficient Serotonin for the task at hand. This last requirement, the call for 5-HTP and its availability to make 5-HT, or serotonin, is regulated by a complex series of unknown processes related to brain activity. As intricate as these processes must be, they occur instantaneously.

Think of it in terms of an extremely sensitive fuel pump in a high tech engine. As the engine increases activity, it calls for more fuel, which the pump responds to by furnishing more fuel; however, in the case of the brain, the pump not only furnishes, but also creates, the fuel. It would be as if your car could manufacture its own gasoline out of raw materials right at the instant it needed fuel. Pretty efficient, these bodies of ours. It was a master engineer who designed us. Can you imagine any other laboratory that could respond this instantaneously by interpreting need, calling up raw material, and then synthesizing the neurotransmitter that stimulates and ignites the action?

Serotonin, or 5-HT, affects the brain in two different ways. First, it has a hormonal effect. The molecules diffuse outward and communicate with other cells, somehow influencing their functioning in a manner we do not completely understand. The second effect, which is better understood, is through the normal action of neurotransmitters.

If the raw material isn't available, the process is going to be slowed and perhaps interrupted completely, and the anticipated "normal" reaction or behavior will not take place. Diets that are deficient in the essential amino acid tryptophan could thus cause some of these abnormalities.

Regulating these steps in the synthesis of Serotonin by the use of psychotropic drugs might be beneficial in treating a variety of deficiency illnesses. Pharmaceutical companies have succeeded in synthesizing drugs that can cause changes in the Serotonin neurotransmission system by either blocking the reuptake of Serotonin at the neuron junction, for example, Prozac and the tricyclic drugs, which intervene in depression, or by inhibiting *enzymes*, biological catalysts, or chemical substances that cause a chemical reaction, without becoming a part of that reaction. This latter category of drugs catalyzes the dissemination of Serotonin. It is not known exactly why and how these drugs biochemically bring about the noticeable behavioral changes.

Although 5-HTP is a safe alternative to serotonin-enhancing drugs, sev eral other compounds that increase serotonin have received some very bad press. The first of these was tryptophan, the amino acid precursor to 5-HTP.

Certain drugs that seem to be effective in treating depression are called the SSRis, which stands for Selective Serotonin Reuptake inhibitors. As their name states, they inhibit the reuptake of Serotonin. This category includes such drugs as Prozac, Paxil, Zoloft, and Luvox. They have caused a revolution in the field of psychiatry. Prior to the invention of Prozac and these other SSRis, psychiatrists had used analysis to deal with severe symptoms of mental disorders, such as psychosis. Now mental health professionals are using a variety of drugs to treat patients for problems that had not normally been treated with medications in the past. These drugs have a very specific method of action, and they are able to relieve symptoms that until now were often considered incurable.

Serotonin cannot cross the blood brain barrier, which means that it cannot leave the bloodstream and pass into the brain tissue, as oxygen and other nutrients do. Therefore, the biosynthesis of brain serotonin necessarily begins in the brain itself. For this reason, it is all the more important to ingest enough tryptophan, or 5-HTP, because the brain cannot take serotonin from other parts of the body that may have sufficient or excess amounts of the neurotransmitter.

One interesting aspect of Serotonin is its structural similarity to a number of hallucinogenic drugs, such as LSD. These hallucinogens seem to partially inhibit the firing of Serotonin neurons by competing with Serotonin at the level of the 5-HT receptors fooling them because they possess a similar chemical structure. The precise biochemical actions of hallucinogenic drugs have not been determined, but their psychological and physiological effects have been studied quite extensively by researchers and fearless, if not foolish, students.

5-HTP Is Safe

Although 5-HTP is a safe alternative to Serotonin-enhancing drugs, several other compounds that increase Serotonin have received some very bad press. The first of these was tryptophan, the amino acid precursor to 5-HTP. During the 1970s and 1980s, this compound was the subject of many studies that found it to be as effective as the tricyclic compounds for treating Serotonin dysfunctions. The tryptophan used in supplements was manufactured in Japan through a process of bacterial fermentation. However, a bad batch of tryptophan, which contained a contaminant, was released by a single Japanese producer. This contaminant caused breakout of a terrible disorder called eosinophilia myalgia syndrome (EMS). As a result, the FDA banned the sale of all tryptophan in the American health food market.

Unlike tryptophan, 5-HTP is not fermented or manufactured through chemical synthesis. It is a natural extract from the seeds of the Grifonia plant.

The other Serotonin enhancers to be removed from the market are fenfluramine and dexflenfluramine (Redux). Fenfluramine, you may remember, was one-half of the popular Fen Phen duo used as an appetite suppressant. When an increase in -the number of people who develop primary pulmonary hypertension was linked to Fenfluramine and Redux use, these two drugs were voluntarily removed from the_ market by their manufacturer. Fenfluramine and Redux are also believed to have caused a rare type of heart valve damage in a small percentage of users. The mechanism involved in these problems has still not been identified and is likely to be unique to these two drugs. No other Serotonin enhancing drug or compound, including the tricyclic antidepressants, the SSRis, the monoamine oxidase inhibitors, or 5-HTP has ever been linked to these types of problems.

Dosing and Precautions for 5-HTP

Since 5-HTP has not had the benefit of pharmaceutical research funding, our knowledge of its safety and efficacy is somewhat sketchy. Though many laboratories and researchers have shown an interest in the chemical, research has not followed a single and organized route. Each lab and researcher has focused on individual interests, and from these many isolated research projects we have tried to glean a comprehensive picture of 5-HTP's characteristics, safety, and benefits. To date, 5-HTP appears to have few side effects and has not shown any remarkable untoward effects in the body.

We would, however, strongly recommend taking certain precautions. If you are under a physician's care for any ailment, and especially if you are already on any type of medication, check with your physician before taking 5-HTP or any other medication, be it prescription or over-the-counter. As an extra precaution, ask your pharmacist's opinion as well. Often, pharmacists are more aware of the dangers of mixing certain medications than physicians are. We also strongly recommend that you buy all of your medications from a single pharmacy so that there is a record in at least one location of every product you use, supervised by an individual who is knowledgeable in the possible effects of combining several drugs and supplements. This is especially important if you go to more than one physician, each of whom may prescribe something without necessarily knowing what other doctors are giving you. It is your responsibility to let all of your health advisers know every remedy you are being treated with.

For example, people who are taking such drugs as Paxil, Zoloft, Prozac, Effexor, and, most especially, MAO inhibitors should exercise caution when considering a regimen of 5-HTP. The result could be an overdose of Serotonin, leading to severe nausea, agitation, lethargy, or any number of unpleasant side effects. Although 5-HTP has few serious side effects when taken alone, it could conceivably trigger serious and lasting side effects of the drugs it is taken with. This has never been observed to happen, so it's a theoretical warning, but it's better to be prudent and avoid the risk.

Supplements of 5-HTP seem to work best when.taken three or more hours after your last meal, especially if the meal was heavy in protein containing foods. Washing 5-HTP down with fruit juice, some people have reported, seems to give it a boost.

The proper dosage should be decided by your physician or pharmacist and may be contingent on other medications or supplements you are taking. The usual dose recommended for sleep seems to be anywhere from 100 to 600 mg at bedtime, a range indicating that people have a very individualized response to the product. It would be wise to start low and increase it upward until you find your ideal dose within the recommended doses.

Quick Review

Let's review the main points of this chapter so that you can come back later to refresh your memory without having to read the whole thing.

Serotonin, or 5-HT, is important in regulating your moods, sleeping, eating, arousal, and dreaming, and it also plays an important role in depression, anxiety, obsessive-compulsive disorders, and numerous other behavior patterns.

Serotonin is not a naturally occurring substance in the diet; it must be synthesized by the body with raw materials that we get from our diet. It is made from the amino acid tryptophan, which is converted into 5-hydroxy-tryptophan, or 5-HTP, by tryptophan hydroxylase, which in turn is converted into 5-HT, or Serotonin.

There are two different ways that 5-H affects the brain. First, it has a hormonal effect. The molecules diffuse outward and communicate with other cells. The second way is through the normal direct action of neurotransmitters.

A category of drugs that are frequently effective in treating depression are called the SSRis, which stands for selective serotonin reuptake inhibitors. As the name states, they inhibit the reuptake of Serotonin and thereby increase its levels in the brain. This category includes such drugs as Prozac, Paxil, Luvox, and Zoloft.

Hopefully, this first chapter hasn't been too boring or intimidating and has given you an idea of how tryptophan, 5-HTP, and serotonin relate to each other and work in your body. I've tried to walk a tightrope between oversimplifying and being overbearing. Our intention is to give us all an equal footing in understanding the body's use of 5-HTP. Now let's move on to discuss the specific processes connected with this product and to examine the intriguing claims that have been made in its name.

DEPRESSION

Carla is a healthy 45-year-old married mother of two. In the past few years, she has complained of fatigue and insomnia and has gained 50 pounds. She used to enjoy outdoor sports with her husband and sons but now no longer wants to leave the house. Her husband feels that Carla doesn't care for her family anymore. He is tired of the frequent arguments Carla picks with the boys and is hurt by her loss of interest in having sex with him. Since her mother's death a few months ago, Carla has started to cry almost daily. "Sometimes I just want to go to sleep and never wake up again."

Carla is suffering from depression and she is not alone. Over 12 million men and women in this country, about 5% of Americans, suffer from some form of depression. The intensity of this depression can range from mildly distressing to severely disabling. Severe depression is a dangerous disease that may lead to death. Over 16,000 people succeed in their suicide at tempts each year.

Depression involves the body, mood, and thoughts. It is all encompassing. It affects the way you eat and sleep, the way you feel about yourself, and how you think about others. A depressive disorder is not a sign of personal weakness or a condition that can be willed or wished away. Those suffering from depression can't just "pull themselves together" and get better. Untreated, symptoms can last for weeks, months, or years. Appropriate treatment, however, can help over 80% of those who suffer from depression.

In the United States the recent treatment of choice for depression has been the selective Serotonin reuptake inhibitors

(SSRis) such as Prozac, Paxil, and Zoloft, as well as other anti depressant drugs such as Effexor, Welbutrin, and Serzone.

Carla's husband finally demanded that she see their doctor for a physical exam. After he diagnosed depression, Carla was surprised that her doctor did not prescribe an antidepressant. She had many friends who took Prozac and other types of SSRis. "I want you try something new," he told her. "It's called 5-HTP and has many of the benefits of traditional antidepressants with none of the side effects." Within two weeks of starting 5-HTP, Carla reported that she was sleeping more and eating less. She had stopped crying and had even lost a few pounds. Four months later her husband reported that she was "back to her old self again." Their sex life improved, to their delight, and she was again hiking with the family.

Depression May Be Due to a Lack of Serotonin

Why did the 5-HTP work so well for Carla? Carla's results with 5-HTP are not uncommon. In fact, the greatest benefit of 5- HTP seems to be in treating depression. As is shown by the success of the SSRis, depression is clearly related to low levels of Serotonin. Taking supplemental 5-HTP may help the body produce more of this essential neurotransmitter.

Researchers investigated this theory when they used a PET scan (positron-emission tomography) to compare the brains of eight healthy volunteers with those of six people diagnosed with major depression. The subjects were given intravenous 5-HTP that was radiolabelled so that the researchers could track its location in the body. They found that there was significantly less 5-HTP in the brains of the depressed subjects than in the brains of the normal controls. The authors concluded that the trans port of 5-HTP into the brain may be compromised in people suffering from major depression.

5-HTP Increases Serotonin Levels

Since a lack of Serotonin appears to be involved in the development of depression, does an increase in 5-HTP actually lead to an increase in serotonin levels? This question was investigated by a group of Japanese researchers. They gave 5-HTP to 24 patients who were hospitalized for depression. Two weeks into treatment, they found a "marked amelioration of depressive symptoms" in seven patients diagnosed with depression. In the subjects' cerebrospinal fluid this team found a 30% increase in the levels of 5-HIAA, a compound formed during the metabolism of Serotonin. Levels of 5-HIAA are commonly used to determine Serotonin levels in humans. This strongly suggested that 5-HTP was being converted to Serotonin and was raising Serotonin levels.

5-HTP Relieves Depressions

But why, then, did Carla's doctor prescribe 5-HTP instead of a "traditional" SSRI? First of all, it works.

In an open study, 25 depressed patients were treated with 5-HTP, either alone or in combination with a peripheral decarboxylase inhibitor, a drug that prevents the body from metabolizing 5-HTP into Serotonin before it can cross into the brain. The researchers found that 5-HTP worked just as well as the traditional antidepressants. The 5-HTP acted quickly within three to five days and produced only minor gastrointestinal side effects. In addition, those who received 5-HTP alone did just as well as those who took the combination, but they had fewer side effects.

In 1987 a study was published that pooled the data on six studies investigating the antidepressive effects of 5HTP. Out of 251 patients, 148 (59%) had a "favorable response" to 5-HTP.

When French researchers treated a group of severely de pressed patients with 5-HTP, they found that 28 of 36 pa tients experienced a lessening of depression. Only four patients felt that there was no benefit and only four could not tolerate the treatment.

5-HTP Relieves Depressions as Well as the SSRis

Although these studies sound impressive, they suffer from one severe weakness: They were open studies. This means that the participants knew they were taking 5-HTP. As has been shown in innumerable studies, the power of suggestion will produce favorable effects in a high percentage of people who know, or falsely believe, that they are taking a real treatment. Thus, the studies described here can't be taken as conclusive.

In order to get around this problem, researchers use what are called "double-blind" studies. In this type of research, some patients are given a treatment while others are given a placebo, and neither doctor nor patient knows which is which. Good results on a properly performed double-blind study can be taken as strong evidence that a treatment really works.

Recently, a double-blind study of the use of 5-HTP to treat depression was performed by a team of Swiss and German psychiatric researchers. Using various standard tests of depression, they compared the effectiveness of 5-HTP and a conventional SSRI. One group of 34 patients received 150 mg of an SSRI that is popular in Europe, fluvoxamine (Luvox), three times a day. The other group of 29 patients received 100 mg of 5-HTP three times a day. Starting at the second week, both groups showed a nearly equal reduction in depression. This neck-and-neck improvement continued through the six weeks of the trial. The improvement in the 5-HTP group was actually slightly better than in the SSRI group by the end, although this difference was not statistically significant. In this study, 5-HTP also improved sleep quality and significantly reduced symptoms of anxiety.

These results are similar to what has been seen in earlier studies that compared the effectiveness of 5-HTP and antidepressant drugs. However, to be realistic, the scientific evidence for 5-HTP's effectiveness must still be regarded as preliminary. The total number of patients in good double-blind studies is still quite small. Until some reasonably large studies are performed, we can't say for certain that we truly know how effective 5-HTP really is.

5-HTP Has Fewer Side Effects Than Reuptake Inhibitors

In the study just described, not only did the 5-HTP work as well as the drug it was compared against, it did so with fewer side effects. Only 14% of the group receiving 5-HTP com plained of side effects, primarily mild digestive distress, and generally most people rated them as "mild" or "very mild."

These symptoms also tended to disappear over the course of the study. In contrast, 18% of the drug group complained of side effects and generally rated them as moderate to severe in intensity. Thus, even though the percentages of side effects are not very different, there was a dramatic difference in the severity of the side effects.

Why did the 5-HTP work so well for Carla? Carla's results with 5-HTP are not uncommon. In fact, the greatest benefits of 5-HTP seems to be in treating depression. As is shown by the success of the SSRis, depression is clearly related to low levels of serotonin. Taking supplemental 5-HTP may help the body produce more of this essential neurotransmitter.

Side effects are a constant problem with conventional antidepressants. Up until the late '80s, the major drugs used to treat depression were in the tricyclic family. These drugs produced many side effects that limited their use, such as daytime sleepiness and lethargy, dry eyes and mouth, dizziness on standing up, and weight gain.

While the modern crop of antidepressants are better, they still frequently cause problems, including nausea, headache, insomnia, agitation, and sexual problems. The most complained-about side effect in women is loss of the ability to experience orgasm. Men sometimes experience impotence, and both sexes may experience loss of libido. Too many men and women have had to make the choice between living de pression free or experiencing a normal sex life. Research has found that taking 5-HTP does not cause this dilemma.

In an evaluation of 17 clinical trials that used 5-HTP, it was concluded that "oral administration of 5-HTP is associated with few adverse effects." The most common side effect is mild digestive distress, and it usually goes away with continued use of the supplement.

How 5-HTP Works

If you recall from the first chapter, Serotonin does not cross the blood-brain barrier. The Serotonin needed for use as a neurotransmitter in the brain must be manufactured in the brain. There are several ways to increase the amount of this serotonin in the brain.

The most popular way is to keep the Serotonin that is already present in the gap between synapses from being removed by the body. After the Serotonin has done its work in the synapse, it is taken up back into the cell. The most popular drugs plug up those take up nozzles so that more Serotonin remains in the gap to continue to do its work.

Another way is to prevent the breakdown of Serotonin. Serotonin is destroyed by an enzyme called monoamine oxidase. By inhibiting this enzyme, more Serotonin becomes available to the neurons. Drugs that work this way are called monoamine oxidase (MAO) inhibitors, but they are rarely used today due to their dangerous side effects.

The third way is to provide more of the raw materials out of which Serotonin is made. Tryptophan can cross the blood-brain barrier and, before its recall, it was used by many practitioners as an alternative to the tricylics and MAO inhibitors. Once inside the brain, tryptophan is changed into 5-HTP and then into Serotonin. An alternative to this is to provide the 5-HTP itself. Since some individuals seem to be unable to easily convert tryptophan into 5-HTP, this is actually a better solution. And, unlike tryptophan, 5-HTP does not have to compete with other amino acids for absorption across the blood-brain barrier. Therefore, 5-HTP is easier to supplement and does not have to be taken in as large a dose as tryptophan.

Double-blind clinical trials that compared the effectiveness of tryptophan and 5-HTP for relieving depression found 5-HTP to be clearly superior. As was mentioned earlier, a few studies have also compared 5-HTP with standard tricyclic antidepressants and found 5-HTP to be at least as effective as these drugs, with fewer side effects.

What Is the Proper Dose of 5-HTP for Depression?

A typical dose of 5-HTP for depression is 100 mg three times a day, starting at 25 or 50 mg and then working up. The full effects take about four weeks to develop, so be patient.

Caution

The fact that 5-HTP can be purchased without a

prescription does not mean that it is a substitute for professional care. Severe depression is too serious an illness for self-treatment. In all cases of significant depression, medical supervision is essential.

Additionally, it is not wise to combine 5-HTP with prescription drug treatment, except on the advice of a qualified health care professional.

Types of Depression

As one might expect, depression can present itself as a feeling of sadness or as "I'm just having the blues." In fact, sadness may not be the most obvious or dominant feeling of a depressed person. Depression can also begin as a numb or empty feeling, or perhaps as an unawareness of feeling. A depressed person may experience a noticeable loss in his or her ability to feel pleasure from anything. Psychiatrists tend to view depression as an illness that causes people to experience a marked change in mood and in the way they view themselves and the world around them. Depression as a significant disorder ranges from that of short duration, to long-term and mild, to very severe and, at worst, life-threatening. Depressive disorders come in different forms, just like other illnesses. The three most prevalent types are major depression, dysthymia, and bipolar disorder.

In the study just described, not only did the 5-HTP work as well as the drug it was compared against, it did so with fewer side effects. Only 14% of the group receiving 5-HTP complained of side effects, primarily mild digestive distress, and generally most people rated them as "mild" or "very mild." These symptoms a/ so tended to disar:r pear over the course of the study. In contrast, 18% of the drug group com plained of side effects and generally rated them as moderate to severe in intensity. Thus, even though the percentages of side effects are not very different, there was a dramatic difference in the severity of the side effects.

Depression and Heart Disease

Certain chronic illnesses are linked to depression. Heart disease, especially post-surgically, more often than not has a very serious depressive phase with it. For example, take the case of David.

David is a 56-year-old stockbroker who describes himself as a workaholic. For two years he has suffered silently from depression and anxiety and recently had a serious heart attack. His cardiologist performed an angioplasty that appears to have removed the blockages in his coronary arteries.

Researchers at the Johns Hopkins University School of Hygiene and Public Health have found that persons who have a history of dysphoria (two weeks of profound sadness), or who have had a major depressive episode, increase their chances of having another heart attack more than four times. This risk was independent of other typical risk factors for heart disease, leading one researcher to comment: "It seems likely that people with heart disease may benefit as much from an antidepressant as from an anti-cholesterol agent."

After his angioplasty was deemed a success, David's doctor treated not only his abnormal lipid levels, but also his depression. David now follows a diet low in saturated fat, rich in fruits and vegetables, and takes 200 mg of 5-HTP each day in divided doses. David's wife has noticed that he no longer buries his problems with work and is more open to share problems with her.

The Diagnosis of Depression

To diagnose true depression, doctors and therapists use the signs and symptoms listed at the end of this chapter, provided that the symptoms have manifested for more than a few weeks and are interfering with the normal living habits of the patient. These signs and symptoms result from an alteration in brain chemistry that is similar to chemical alterations that can cause Depression be triggered by any illness, stress, frustration, or grief. It differs, however, in that it is self-sustaining, not resolving itself upon removal of the triggering event if and when the causative event or situation can be found and alleviated.

While the modern crop of antidepressants are better, they still frequently cause problems, including nausea, headache, insomnia, agitation, and sexual problems. The most complained-about side effect in women is loss of the ability to experience orgasm. Men sometimes experience impotence, and both sexes may experience loss of libido. Too many men and women have had to make the choice between living depression free or experiencing a normal sex life. Research has found that taking 5-HTP does not cause this dilemma.

Instead, the alteration continues beyond the effectiveness of the triggering situation, often producing progressively worse symptoms of depression and morbid feelings. Furthermore, those symptoms often inflict additional intense stresses on the person, resulting in new and more severe symptoms, growing unhappiness, sleep disorders, lack of concentration, difficulty doing one's job, and an inability to care for one's own physical and emotional needs, which cause increased strain on relationships with friends, fellow workers, and family. Frequently, these new stresses may be sufficiently acute to act as triggers for continuing brain chemistry alteration, which prevents the resolution of the difficulties that may have triggered the initial alteration, or both. Coping becomes more and more difficult, as the cycle devolves into even deeper depression. If Serotonin deficiency is one of the chemical changes in this cycle, then theoretically 5-HTP could be beneficial in the interruption of the downward spiral.

This brain chemistry alteration should be self-limiting in most cases, but without treatment the resolution of the imbalance can be very slow, taking one to three years before a more normal chemistry returns. A serious danger in waiting for depression to run its course is that if the alteration is profound enough to cause suicidal impulses, a majority of untreated depressed people will attempt suicide, and up to 20% will eventually succeed. Frequently, the untreated depressed patient will try suicide not really to end life but, rather, as a cry for help. All too often that cry for help goes wrong and ends in a tragic death. Any form of depression must be considered a potentially fatal illness. *Never be deceived by the casual way that profoundly depressed people speak of suicide or self-mutilation, especially in the case of children and teenagers.* It's not that they are being casual because they don't really mean it and are making idle threats in order to get attention they are casual In the way they talk about death because suicide seems no worse than the mental pain they are already suffering. Whenever a depressed person of any age speaks of suicide or seems to dwell on death or shows an inclination toward self-mutilation, that person must be taken to a professional for intervention and help. If the per son is already under professional care, his or her comments or actions must be brought to the attention of that professional immediately. If the professional seems casual or unworried about the situation, change to another professional.

There is no such thing as a depressed person making an idle threat of suicide!

Depression often short-circuits the survival instinct or temporarily suppresses it. Therefore, depressed suicidal thinking is not the same as the suicidal thinking of normal people who have reached a crisis point in their lives. Depressive suicides give less warning, need less time to plan, and are willing to attempt more painful and immediate means, such as jumping out of a moving car or a high window or into traffic. They may also fight the impulse to kill themselves by compromising with committing violent mutilation and serious, permanent self injury, cutting themselves with knives or amputating body parts in an attempt to distract themselves from severe mental pain. Again, relatives and friends are likely to be astonished by how quickly such an impulse can be acted upon.

Clinical Depression

So just how do we know when the emotions we are experiencing are simply our normal response to "a bad hair day" or symptoms and signs of something much more serious? Major all, ups and downs are always with us. How can we tell if our normal sad response is just that, or if are we indeed headed into a more serious situation? The transitions from a bad hair day to "I'm getting into a real rut" to full-blown clinical depression can be very small.

In later chapters we will discuss the role of 5-HTP in the treatment of sleep disorders, to counteract pain, in appetite suppression, and for several other problems that can add to the distress of a depressed person. Merely by relieving the other factors that complicate the overall depression syndrome, 5-

HTP might make a tremendous difference in helping a depressed patient cope with the myriad of problems he or she faces.

Clinical depression is a medical illness that even the strongest person can rarely overcome without treatment. All of us have a susceptibility to it, as we do to any other physical disease. If we have a family history of depression, our susceptibility increases. This explains how some people develop clinical depression only after extraordinary stressors, while others develop clinical depression with seemingly little previously noticed stress or cause. Clinical depression is a very common illness that affects approximately 3% to 5% of our population at any given time. The average person has a 20% chance of undergoing an episode of clinical depression at some point in his or her life. Being clinically depressed, as the symptoms listed at the end of the chapter suggest, is very different from having the low and sad feelings we all experience from time to time. Occasional feelings of sadness are a normal part of life, and it is in most cases an overstatement to call them "depression."

In clinical depression, one's despondent feelings are out of proportion to any obvious external cause. "Incapacity" is the defining factor. People who are not clinically depressed manage to cope with the worst problems without becoming incapacitated. The clinically depressed person can't seem to cope with even minor setbacks.

Women are more than twice as likely as men to experience a major depressive episode. Women produce more melatonin during the winter than during summer months. Men produce melatonin at the same rate year-round. Melatonin is a hormone that is made from 5-HTP.

Dysthymia

Dysthymia is a less severe depression; it manifests through long-term, chronic symptoms that are not, however, completely disabling. Dysthymia keeps the patient from functioning at full capacity or from feeling up to par. Sometimes people with dysthymia go in and out of more acute depressive episodes.

Postpartum Depression

Anxiety and mild moodiness are quite common after the delivery of a baby, but when these symptoms become more than just mild anxiety over new responsibilities and depression begins to overwhelm the normal maternal instincts and feelings and lasts longer than just a few days, the serious problem of postpartum depression may be developing. In more than a few cases, this will occur after the mother's discharge from the hospital, to the consternation of the family who expected only joy over the new addition to the household. The cause for this type of depression is thought to be hormonal in etiology, although it may have numerous stress triggers. Since postpartum depression can occur after the birth of any child, even if the mother has previously given birth to other children without becoming depressed, it is obvious that the stress of having a newborn is unlikely to be a major causative factor. Probably, more important factors are the mother's age and the way pregnancy affects her hormonal balance and her subsequent recovery.

Dr. Lotter is a naturopathic physician in Santa Barbara, California. She recalls a woman who came to her with postpartum depression. 'The only thing that would help was Prozac. I worked with her medical doctor to wean her off Prozac and onto 5-HTP. Not only did she have no appetite, but she had no sex drive. Now she is doing really well and her sex drive has returned to normal."

Although mothers suffering from this type of depression usually discontinue nursing, 5-HTP should not be taken without their doctor's knowledge since there are no studies showing the effect of 5-HTP on lactation or on infants and children.

Professional help should be sought as soon as the symptoms of postpartum depression are suspected, since postpartum depression can be extremely serious and dangerous for both mother and baby. Self mutilation and suicide, as well as serious harm and mortal injury to the baby, are not uncommon in critical cases of postpartum depression.

The severity of postpartum depression is related to the level of tryptophan in the blood. The lowest tryptophan levels were seen in the women having the most severe depressions.

The Tendency for Depression to Be Inherited

The brain chemistry of certain people seems to be more predisposed to a depressive chemical response than the brain chemistry of others, who appear to have a much lower risk of depression even when they are exposed to the same or far greater physical or psychological distress or triggers. The genetic relatives of manic-depressives are at a considerably higher risk for unipolar depression than the population at large. Furthermore, since individuals who enter, by either adoption or marriage, into a family with a history of depression are not necessarily more prone to the disease than the general population, this indicates a genetic predisposition. If this genetic predisposition is due to the way the brain uses and metabolizes chemical links and neurotransmitters, then a supplemental or medicinal treatment should be strongly considered. Prescribing 5-HTP might be beneficial in such genetic cases.

There is also an interesting creative factor involved in bipolar, or manic-depressive, disease. Few people doubt the apparent link that exists between high creativity and the gene for manic depression. An inordinate number of artists, actors, sculptors, and writers, if not bipolar themselves, have close family members who are. Studies of families that had members of each generation developing manic-depressive illnesses found that those with the illness have a somewhat different genetic make-up than those who do not show signs of bipolar disease. However, not everyone with the genetic make-up that causes vulnerability to manic depressive disease has the disorder, indicating that additional factors, such as a stressful environment, are involved in the fulmination of the disease.

Other major types of depression also seem to occur in the same families, generation after generation. Nonetheless, we should not feel a false sense of security if no one in our family is known to have been depressive. Depression can occur in people who have no family history of any form of mental illness. No human being is entirely immune to depression or any other form of mental illness under all possible conditions. Some of us cope better than others, but we all have our limits and no one can predict where our threshold lies or how close we are to approaching it. Perhaps when stresses are too great, a product such as 5-HTP would be a better and safer prophylactic than the strong and addictive tranquilizers we too often have prescribed for ourselves and our loved ones.

Psychological Triggers

Virtually all of us can point to some incident or condition that is responsible for our occasional unhappiness and serious distress. Fortunately, most of the time we can cope with our sadness and disappointments. People with severe depression are prone to astonishingly virulent and inappropriate guilt and self-hatred when dour events disrupt their otherwise ordered lives.

Drastic life crises that most often trigger depression are many and varied, but there is one distinguishing feature that appears in most cases, *loss*, whether it be loss of empowerment, of self-confidence, of self-determination, or of control over one's destiny. More profoundly, there is a loss of self-identity, a loss of the abilities that a person identifies with him, or herself. A man loses the job or profession that had defined him to himself and others, "executive" or "breadwinner," "man of the house," "head of the family." A woman who had spent her whole life preparing for and living the role of wife, supporter, and caretaker is suddenly left alone through the divorce or death of her spouse and, as a result, feels she no longer has a purpose. Any normal or unexpected lifecycle change, or any change caused by events beyond your control, changes that damage the structure that invested your life with meaning, can plunge you into deep, debilitating depression.

A person's ability to cope in such an event will depend on many factors, including genetic predisposition, support from friends, physical health, environment, other stresses occurring at the time, the season of the year, and even the weather. It can also depend on internal psychological factors that may best be explored in talk therapy: Why is the person's self-esteem so bound up in the position or state that has been lost? Can she find a new source of self-esteem and purpose?

Of course, not everyone who is victim to this sort of event becomes depressed, and not all people who become depressed have had this sort of catastrophe befall them. A person may suffer a loss and become normally saddened, may grieve, may feel a normal amount of depressed feelings, and may weather the loss in fine style-and then succumb to a much less obvious trigger, whether psychological, physical, or chemical. Some depressions may well be caused by a spontaneous aberration in the brain chemistry, perhaps brought on by a seizure or a migraine or some illness or fever that *may* be a trigger but they are not a trigger that we can currently identify; thus, the subsequent depression appears to be spontaneous. However, once the depressive state has set in, both physical and psychological problems will be generated in abundance. What faster way is there to lose a job or a spouse or a home than to be too depressed to work or to communicate? What can be worse for self-esteem than watching one's household and life goals disintegrate? When health begins to deteriorate as well, recovery becomes all the more difficult. Erratic eating habits can cause high carbohydrate and low protein induced Serotonin imbalance, further complicating the chemistry of the depressive state. Almost no one has the impulse to exercise or get fresh air and sunshine. All of these effects can form feedback loops, increasing in magnitude and becoming triggers for further depression.

The question "Is depression mostly physical or psychological?" is rather beside the point. Depression may be triggered by either physical or psychological events, but once triggered it feeds on itself. Most commonly, both psychology and physiology (or pathology) are involved and it is difficult to separate the two when one is talking about psychology and neurochemistry. However it begins, depression quickly develops into a set of physical and psychological problems that feed on each other, spiral, and grow. A simple match may start a fire, but its eventual destructive force will depend on what fuels it. This is why a combination of physical and psychological interventions has been shown to give the best results for most patients, regardless of any classifications that doctors may impose on the depression and its cause.

Researchers at the Johns Hopkins University School of Hygiene and Public Health have found that persons who have a history of dysphoria (two weeks of profound sadness), or who have had a major depressive episode, increase their chances of having another heart attack more than four times. This risk was independent of other typical risk factors for heart disease, leading one researcher to comment: "It seems likely that people with heart disease may benefit as much from an antidepressant as from an anti-cholesterol agent."

How Treatable Is Clinical Depression?

Clinical depression is readily treatable with counseling and/or medication. Medication can correct the chemical imbalance, such as low levels of brain Serotonin and other mediators and neurotransmitters, that is found in people having symptoms consistent with clinical depression. Unfortunately, over half the people who have clinical depression never get help and suffer silently. Untreated, the average clinical depression can last six months to a year or longer. With treatment, people often report significant relief within a few weeks.

If you or a friend or loved one have symptoms suggestive of any form of depression, seek professional help. Communicate your feelings freely. If you are uncomfortable with the help you are getting, seek new counsel until you find a professional you trust and can confide in comfortably. Discuss your treatment so that you know what its goals and principles are. Feel free to question what you doubt or don't understand. Your thoughts and feelings are important to your treatment and recovery. Ask about all of the medications you take so that you understand their purpose, their side effects, and their hoped-for effects.

In later chapters we will discuss the role of 5-HTP in the treatment of sleep disorders, to counteract pain, in appetite suppression, and for several other problems that can add to the distress of a depressed person. Merely by relieving the other factors that complicate the overall depression syndrome, 5-HTP might make a tremendous difference in helping a depressed patient cope with the myriad of problems he or she faces.

We've all had bad days, even really bad days when nothing seemed to go right and we became more and more depressed as the day dragged on. That one bad day may even have turned into several bad days or a miserable week. Sound familiar? Perhaps you lost a job or went through a nasty divorce, lost a loved one or lost material possessions through some mishap. Mishaps and tragedies happen to all of us, and it is only natural to respond with sadness, even with some really depressed feelings.

What Are the Signs of Severe Clinical Depression?

• Your concentration is impaired.

You can't keep your mind on anything you're doing. Your thoughts keep drifting back to your feelings of hopelessness and how bad things are.

• You seem to be unable to experience pleasure.

Even things that always gave you great pleasure now don't even raise your interest. You seem to care about noth ing and can only dwell on your misery.

• You have thoughts of self-depreciation.

You continually make harsh, negative statements about yourself. You wonder how anyone could possibly even like you.

• You suffer from sleep disturbances or are unable to fall back to sleep.

You can't escape your depression by finding peaceful rest.

Even when you do manage to doze, it is fitful and unsatisfying.

• You have feelings of fatigue even after sleep.

If you do finally fall asleep out of sheer exhaustion, you wake up still fatigued, even after long hours of deep sleep.

• You have a marked decrease in appetite.

You find that food seems to have lost its taste. Even favorite foods no longer interest you.

• You develop strong feelings of guilt, helplessness, and, above all, hopelessness.

Even when others try to convince you that things aren't that bad, you may grasp it intellectually but not emotionally.

• You may entertain thoughts of suicide.

These self-destructive impulses may be fleeting, or you may even go so far as to start planning how you would do it. You may see suicide as your only solution, the only way out.

• You begin to isolate yourself.

For days you don't want to see another person. You just want to stay in bed so that you don't have to see or talk to anyone.

• You lose interest in your responsibilities.

You begin to miss deadlines and lower your work standards. You neglect your bills and obligations to others.

• Your friends notice a change in your personality.

They begin to mention that you've changed, or worse, they start to avoid you. You don't really seem to care.

• You go to extremes sexually.

You either lose all interest in sex or you may increase your sexual activity, perhaps even to the point of promiscuity. Your sexual personality may change from gentle and considerate to rough and hedonistic.

• You may increase your alcohol and tobacco consumption or turn to drug use.

You are in danger of becoming addicted, especially to mind-altering drugs-either prescription or illicit.

• You have feelings of hopelessness, pessimism.

You become pessimistic to the extreme of believing that nothing will ever go your way again and that everything is hopeless, even life itself.

• You experience appetite loss with accompanying rapid weight loss, or else massive overeating and weight gain.

Your loss of appetite and distaste for food may take a radical turn and you may become glutton.

• You have decreased energy and suffer from extreme fatigue.

You just don't have the energy to do anything unless you are absolutely forced to. You procrastinate and seem to lose all sense of priority. Nothing seems important.

• You are restless and irritable.

The previously mentioned extreme fatigue may be interspersed with brief periods of restlessness and intense irritability, but these do not bring about any real productive effort.

• You have difficulty remembering things and making decisions.

You can't make decisions about even the simplest mat ters and tend to forget things that would normally be important to you.

• You have persistent physical symptoms.

You develop minor ailments that do not respond to treatment, such as headaches, digestive disorders, and chronic pain. You become hypersensitive to symptoms that would normally not cause concern, you tend toward hypochondria. Conversely, you may lose all interest in your health status.

• You neglect common hygiene.

You become unkempt; care not whether you bathe; be come unconcerned with the cleanliness of your body, your clothing, or your environment; and may go for days without changing from your bed clothing or without shaving or using make-up.

If you or someone you know experiences even a few of these signs and symptoms for more than two weeks, there is a good chance that severe clinical depression is the cause. Professional help should be sought at once.

ANXIETY AND PANIC DISORDERS

Mary is a graduate student in her mid-20s. She has always described herself as a worrier, but in the past year she finds it more and more difficult to separate herself from her school work. She constantly finds herself thinking and worrying about her grades and her future. During her last physical exam, Mary told her doctor that she "felt jumpy all the time," did not sleep well at night, and was having trouble concentrating on her studies. Her doctor noted that her heart rate and pulse were rapid, her hands and feet were cold, and her muscles were tense. Mary's physician diagnosed an anxiety disorder.

What is the difference between anxiety, or worry, and panic? According to University of Illinois psychologist Wendy Heller, "worry seems to be associated more with verbal ruminating, obsessing, or making up stories in your head. Panic is much more a physiological state of alertness in which a person responds to a perceived threat with heart pounding, hands sweating, light-headedness, and/or dizziness."

Anxiety is as much a part of everyone's life as are laughter and tears, happiness and disappointment, and eating and sleeping. In fact, anxiety is present almost every day of our lives, and in most cases it is essential and beneficial as a motivator and as protection. It piques our attention, our alertness, and readies our minds and bodies for action. Challenged by new and unfamiliar situations, we are spurred by anxiety to meet the test. Stage fright provides us with the best motivation to practice and prepare for a presentation or recital. And that same anxiety, or fear, urges us to react or flee when faced with threat or danger. Anxiety, then, under normal conditions, can be a strong motivator as well as a protection from danger.

As we can see from Mary's case, anxiety and fear are not normal when they become overwhelming and interfere with normal daily living patterns. Then they are symptoms of an anxiety disorder, the most common form of mental illness. Fortunately, anxiety disorders also have the best prognosis for successful treatment.

Anxiety disorders afflict up to 20% of Americans during any given year, and such disorders will affect virtually all of us at one or more times in our lives. Most episodes are transient and often self-limiting. Think back and you will probably recall a time when some threatening circumstance became so overwhelming that it took possession of you, to the point that you could not cope and were unable to attend to other obligations and responsibilities.

The Physiology of Anxiety

Scientists believe that anxiety and panic result from complex electrochemical interactions in the aut0nomic nervous system, the branch of your nervous system that acts without being under the conscious control of the brain. During periods of perceived stress, the adrenal glands increase their secretion of adrenaline and cortisol. This is often called the fight or flight response. These hormones are responsible for the classic symptoms of anxiety: racing heart and pulse, cold and clammy hands and feet, tight muscles, and rapid shallow breathing.

What is the difference between anxiety, or worry, and panic? According to University of Illinois psychologist Wendy Heller, "worry seems to be associated more with verbal ruminating, obsessing, or making up stories in your head. Panic is much more a physiological state of alertness in which a person responds to a perceived threat with heart pounding, hands sweating, light-headedness, and/or dizziness."

Researchers at Johns Hopkins believe they have even identified the location in the brain where worrying takes place. Using PET scans that measure blood-flow variations, the scientists concluded that several structures on the right side are the site of anxious thoughts. 'We saw an increase in the right frontal lobe, the planning and decision-making part of the brain, and in other areas on the right that are involved in arousal, self-examination, and processing of new inputs," Hoehn-Saric, one of the researchers, explained. The other areas included the basal ganglia, which coordinate and process messages from various parts of the brain; the cerebellum, whose functions include storing routines frequently used patterns of thought or movements; and the pontine nuclei, which regulate arousal.

University of Illinois researchers reported similar results. They found that panic attacks during times of environmental stress are accompanied by increased electrical activity in the right posterior of the brain. While at rest, worriers showed more activity in the left frontal section.

According to the journal *Science*, Drs. Klaus-Peter Lesch and Armin Heils of the University of Wurzburg believe they have found the gene responsible for anxiety. This gene encodes a transporter protein that aids Serotonin uptake (Serotonin is regarded as an anxiety modulator). One variant of the gene leads to more Serotonin, while another variant leads to less. This may explain why drugs that increase the levels of Serotonin are often effective in reducing anxiety. The high cortisol levels produced by anxiety also reduce the level of Serotonin in the brain. In animal experiments, prolonged exposure to cortisol has even been shown to damage the serotonin producing nerves in the brain.

Let's return to Mary's story.

Mary's anxiety was starting to take over her life. She was even thinking of dropping out of graduate school. Her doctor recommended a stress reduction class to teach her to deal with her anxieties, along with vitamin and mineral supplementation and a trial of 5-HTP. One year later Mary reports that she now sleeps through the night, that her anxiety has disappeared, and that her concentration has greatly improved. Mary plans to graduate this year.

If Mary's doctor were less holistically inclined, she would have suggested a more pharmacological approach to Mary's anxiety disorder, such as Xanax, Buspar, or an SSRI. These Serotonin-enhancing drugs have been shown to relieve anxiety. But Mary's doctor was also familiar with a body of preliminary research suggesting that 5-HTP can also be effective.

• Ten patients diagnosed with anxiety syndromes were treated with 5-HTP. Using three different scales designed to mea sure anxiety, researchers found a significant reduction in anxiety.

• Another study of 20 people with panic disorders found that several experienced a feeling of "relief' after receiving 5-HTP.

These studies cannot be taken as proof that 5-HTP is effective. However, if 5-HTP can treat depression, there is every reason to expect it should be useful for anxiety as well. Virtually all prescription antidepressants can be used in the treatment of anxiety, for reasons that are not at all clear.

What Is the Proper Dosage of 5HTP for Anxiety?

Supplemental 5-HTP may be used in the same dose at which it is used to treat depression, 100 mg three times daily, with meals.

Caution:

Severe anxiety can be a terrible, disabling disease. Because the true effectiveness rate of 5-HTP in anxiety isn't yet known, it certainly can't be counted on to provide sure relief. Medical supervision is essential.

Additionally, it is not wise to combine 5-HTP with prescription drug treatment, except on the advice of a qualified health care professional.

Types of Anxiety Disorders

Anxiety is such a commonly used word that it loses its impact for many people, who don't realize what anxiety means in mental health terms and just how devastating it can be. Further complicating matters is the fact that *anxiety* and *fear* are often used to describe the same feeling when, in fact, they are not exactly synonymous. When the word *anxiety* is used to discuss a group of mental illnesses, it should refer to a specific disease process with an identifiable cause. The word *fear*, on the other hand, should refer to the cause of a mental tension that is due to a specific external threat, such as when an unfriendly dog shows his intent by growling and baring his fangs at you.

"Anxiety disorders" thus refer to a group of illnesses subcategorized into: generalized anxiety disorders, phobias, panic disorders, post-traumatic stress disorders, and obsessive-compulsive disorders. These sub-groupings are more descriptive of the symptoms of the form the individual's anxiety takes.

Generalized Anxiety Disorder

People with generalized anxiety disorder suffer from unrealistic worries and fears about every aspect of life. They may worry about financial matters even though they have a more-than-adequate bank balance and have paid their debts in full. They may be constantly preoccupied about the welfare of a child or other loved one who is safe at school or at home. People with generalized anxiety disorder may have stretches of time when they're not consumed by these worries, but they are anxious most of the time. Patients with this disorder often feel "uneasy," "keyed up," or "on edge," and they sometimes "go blank" because of the tension that they feel. Often they also suffer from a degree of depression.

Panic Disorders

Susan is 58 years old, with a predisposition to anxiety. In her early 50s she had developed panic disorder and twice had become dependent on Xanax. When Susan came to her doctor, she wanted to improve her life overall and one of things she wanted was to resolve her panic disorder. Her physician recommended 5-HTP. As long as Susan remains on 5-HTP, she has no anxiety.

These studies cannot be taken as proof that 5-HTP is effective. However, if 5-HTP can treat depression, there is every reason to expect it should be useful for anxiety as well. Virtually all prescription antidepressants can be used in the treatment of anxiety, for reasons that are not at all clear.

Panic disorders afflict up to 3 million Americans each year. Victims suddenly suffer intense, overwhelming terror for no apparent reason. The fear is accompanied by at least four of the following symptoms: profuse sweating; fierce trembling; heart palpitations; feelings of unreality; hot or cold flashes; blushing or pallor; choking, smothering sensations, or feeling a lump in the throat; shortness of breath; chest and breathing discomfort; faintness; vertigo; fear of losing control of one's actions, of dying, or of losing one's mind and going crazy; unsteadiness; or tingling and weakness of the limbs.

Often, people suffering from a panic attack for the first time rush to the hospital, convinced they are having a heart attack or a stroke and that death is at the doorstep. Attacks can't be predicted and can occur at the least expected times; paradoxically, they are not necessarily brought on during stressful times. Certain situations, however, such as driving a car, can become associated with a feeling of panic if that was the situation in which the first attack occurred. Untreated, panic sufferers can become suicidal.

Phobias

This type of anxiety disorder afflicts up to 15% of all Americans during their lifetimes. People who suffer from this illness feel terror, dread, or panic when confronted with the feared object, situation, or activity, and they cannot give a reasonable explanation for why they fear the object of their dread. Many have such an overwhelming desire to avoid the source of their fear that it interferes with their jobs, family life, and social relationships. They may lose their jobs because they can't go to business lunches for fear of eating in front of others. They may quit a job in a high-rise office in order to work on the ground floor because they fear elevators. They may become so fearful of leaving their homes that they live like hermits.

Obsessive-Compulsive Disorders

Karen is a successful screenwriter. During periods of stress, Karen pulls out her hair, a condition called trichotillomania. Only Paxil prevented this behavior until Karen discovered 5-HTP. As long as Karen takes her 5-HTP, she does not engage in this behavior and feels less stressed and anxious.

Obsessive-compulsive disorders (OCD) afflict 2.5 million Americans. People with OCD suffer from obsessional behaviors, which are repeated, intrusive, unwanted thoughts and actions that cause distress and extreme anxiety. They may also suffer from compulsive behaviors that psychiatrists define as ritualistic , such as hand-washing, repeated actions like relocking a door a given number of times, rechecking something several times over to make sure it's as it should be in an attempt to reduce their irrational anxiety about something that is usually inconsequential. People who suffer from obsessive disorders do not necessarily perform compulsive behaviors, but most do have obsessions. Victims of obsessions are plagued with persistent, frightening, involuntary thoughts or impulses, such as fearing they will become infected by shaking hands with others. These thoughts can be fleeting and momentary, or they can be lasting ruminations.

People with compulsions may go through senseless, repeated, and involuntary ritualistic behaviors that they believe will prevent or bring about a future event. However, the rituals themselves have nothing to do with the anticipated event. For example, a person may constantly wash his or her hands or touch a particular object in hopes that it will ward off some expected disaster. Often, people with this disorder also suffer from a complementary obsession such as worry over contracting an infection.

Examples of compulsive rituals include: cleaning over and over and over, which affects women more often than men, and if the patients come in contact with any dirt, they may spend hours washing and cleaning, even to the point that their hands bleed. They may repeat a behavior, such as saying a loved one's name several times whenever that person comes up in conversation. Checking things over and over repeatedly tends to affect men more than women. For example, patients check and recheck that doors are locked or that electric switches, gas ovens, and water taps are turned off. Other patients will retrace a route they have driven in order to check that they did not hit a pedestrian or cause an accident without knowing it. The activities are not at all rational to the observer.

There is reason for optimism about treatment of even the most severe anxiety disorders. Research indicates that 65% to 75% of the phobic and obsessive patients who can cooperate with the therapist and conscientiously follow instructions will recover with behavior therapy. Studies have shown that while they are taking the medications, 70% of the patients who suffer from panic attacks improve. Medication is effective for about half of those suffering from obsessive-compulsive disorder.

The biochemical basis of obsessive-compulsive disorder has not yet been clarified. Drugs that increase Serotonin, such as the SSRis, decrease the compulsive behavior and anxiety in about one-half of those who take them.

Obsessive-compulsive disorders often begin during the teens or early adulthood. Generally, they are chronic and cause moderate to severe disability in their victims. They do not usually lead to suicidal or hostile actions.

Post-Traumatic Stress Disorder

Post-traumatic stress disorder (PTSD) is a form of depression most often associated with war veterans and was called shell shock after World Wars I and II. But post-traumatic stress disorder can occur in anyone who has experienced a severe and unusual physical or mental trauma. People who have witnessed a midair collision or survived rape or a life-threatening crime may develop this illness. The severity of the disorder increases if the trauma was unanticipated. For that reason, not all war veterans develop PTSD, despite prolonged and brutal combat. Soldiers expect a certain amount of violence. Rape victims, however, are unsuspecting of the attack on their bodies and lives and may suffer PTSD even more severely than a battle-weary soldier.

People who suffer from PTSD re-experience the event that traumatized them through frightening and realistic night mares, night terrors, or flashbacks of the event. In rare cases, the person falls into a temporary dislocation from reality in which he or she relives the trauma. This can last from a few terrifying seconds to horribly agonizing days. "Psychic numbing," or emotional anesthesia, occurs when victims have de creased interest in, or involvement with, people or activities they once enjoyed. The patient may suffer from excessive alertness and highly sharpened senses and an exaggerated startle reaction. A car backfiring may cause people who were once subjected to gunfire to instinctively drop to the ground or go into hysterics.

Trauma victims with PTDS suffer from general anxiety, depression, inability to sleep, poor memory, and difficulty concentrating on or completing tasks; they often have severe survivor's guilt, which can lead to suicide.

Theories About Causes
of Anxiety Disorders

Probably no single situation or condition causes anxiety disorders; rather, physical and environmental triggers may combine to create a particular anxiety illness. Psychoanalytic theory sug gests that anxiety stems from unconscious conflicts that arose from discomfort during infancy or childhood. The person may have developed problems from experiencing an illness, fright, or other emotionally laden event as a child. According to this theory, anxiety can be resolved by identifying and resolving or defusing the unconscious conflict so that symptoms symbolizing the conflict would then disappear.

Learning theory says that anxiety is a learned behavior that can be unlearned. People who feel uncomfortable in a given situation or near a certain object can train themselves to lessen the threat, accept the threat, or learn to avoid it. However, such avoidance can limit a patient's ability to live a normal life.

Treatments

Generally, anxiety disorders are treated by a combination approach. Phobias and obsessive-compulsive disorders are often treated with behavior therapy. This involves exposing the patient to the feared object or situation under controlled circumstances, until the fear is cured or significantly reduced. Successfully treated with this method, many phobia patients have long-term recovery. Medications are effective treatments, sometimes used alone and often in combination with behavior therapy or other psychotherapy techniques.

There is reason for optimism about treatment of even the most severe anxiety disorders. Research indicates that 65% to 75% of the phobic and obsessive patients who can cooperate with the therapist and conscientiously follow instructions will recover with behavior therapy. Studies have shown that while they are taking the medications, 70% of the patients who suffer from panic attacks improve. Medication is effective for about half of those suffering from obsessive-compulsive disorder.

Symptoms Frequently Associated with Severe Anxiety

• Unrealistic or excessive worry

We all have worries. Most are justified, even though many of the things we worry about never come to pass, yet it is still perfectly normal to worry about them. The pessimists among us worry more than the optimists, but neither type of person is more or less normal than the other. Nevertheless, when worry is the predominant emotion in our lives, then it becomes abnormal. If a person cannot enjoy or look forward to anything without having so much concern that it tortures him or her, then this is abnormal. If you are convinced beyond reason that absolutely nothing can go right, then your anxiety is out of balance.

• Exaggerated startle reactions

If the doorbell or phone ringing causes an adrenaline rush and gets you upset, that is a far cry from jumping when some one unexpectedly bursts a balloon and causes you to react. Overreaction once in a while is quite within normal limits, but when overreaction becomes your norm, that's not normal.

• Sleep disturbances

Who hasn't had a sleepless night over some specific problem? But when you can't get a sound sleep for several nights in a row, tossing restlessly even when you doze, or when you can't stay asleep more than a few minutes or an hour without awakening to your worries and fears, then your anxieties are out of control.

• Tremulousness, shakes, and muscle aches

Sometimes a sudden scare leaves us with the "shakes," but when the shakes go on for hours at a time, to the point that they cause muscle spasms and pain, you are probably in need of professional help to reverse the physical reaction to your anxiety.

• Cold and clammy hands, the sweats, hot flashes, and inter mittent chills.

These are responses to the "fight or flight" neurotransmitters, the "adrenaline rush" and its aftermath. Like the tremors, they may require temporary tranquilization. But don't be satisfied with tranquilization that does not include an effort to seek and treat the cause of your anxiety.

• Fatigue

The fatigue that comes with anxiety can be due to lack of sleep, poor sleep, the hyperactivity that often accompanies anxiety, the constant dwelling on problems real or imagined, tremors, or any number of other symptoms. Some of these causes of fatigue are due to the adrenaline-like neurotransmitters and some are mediated by Serotonin. Supplemental 5-HTP might be helpful as an adjunct to treatment, but make sure you discuss it with your physician or pharmacist, especially if you are on tranquilizers or other medications.

The fatigue that comes with anxiety can be due to lack of sleep, poor sleep, the hyperactivity that often accompanies anxiety, the constant dwelling on problems real or imagined, tremors, or any number of other symptoms.

Some of these causes of fatigue are due to the adrenaline-like neurotransmitters and some are mediated by serotonin. Supplemental 5-HTP might be helpful as an adjunct to treatment, but make sure you discuss it with your physician or pharmacist, especially if you are on tranquilizers or other medications.

• Drymouth

Dryness of the mouth could be brought on by the adrenaline effects of anxiety or it could be due to medication. Call it to the attention of your physician or pharmacist. Chewing gum, eating lozenges or candy, or increasing your intake of fluids may take care of the problem.

• Unrealistic fears concerning certain objects or situations

When you start to fear normally harmless situations and objects, or start assigning powers and personalities to them, you are on the verge of hallucinations and paranoia. Professional help is needed. By this time, the patient is not in a position to realize his or her need, and friends and relatives will have to intervene.

• "Flashbacks" of past trauma and terrors

In World Wars I and II, it was called "shell shock"; today it is called "post-traumatic stress syndrome." Flashbacks also occur to people who have been part of the drug culture and who may relive a "bad trip." These are vivid experiences, with all the terror of the past experiences. Some patients will tell you the flashback is much worse than the original or actual experience ever was. Intensive treatment is usually required. Yet 5-HTP may be helpful as a supplementary therapy.

• Ritualistic behaviors

Often patients with long-standing anxiety deal with their apprehensions by performing elaborate ritualistic behaviors. Remember Macbeth and the ritualistic hand-washing, as an attempt to deal with the anxiety caused by guilt? This ritualistic behavior may be closely related to the cause of the anxiety, or it may be very bizarre, with significance only in the subconscious mind of the patient.

• Racing or pounding heart

Palpitations are very common in anxiety, almost the rule-just like the pounding of your heart when someone or something scares you. It is usually part of the adrenaline effect. It can be very annoying but is usually not dangerous unless you have an underlying heart problem. It should be mentioned to your physician. It often adds to your anxiety, and relieving your fear of it can be helpful.

• Numbness and tingling of the hands, feet, or other body parts

This is often related to hyperventilation and is scary but not often dangerous, unless it occurs while you are in a vulnerable situation such as driving or walking on stairs or in a place where you might fall into dangerous surroundings or equipment. Breathing into a paper bag will usually resolve the problem; or, if you can, make yourself hold your breath for as long as possible, take a few slow breaths, and then hold your breath again. This last maneuver is difficult for someone having terrors.

• Upset stomach

Abdominal pain, indigestion, and digestive problems often accompany anxiety. Avoidance of high-fat diets and excessive spices can help. Taking small portions more fre quently and the use of antacids may be beneficial. If the upset stomach persists for more than two or three days, no tify your doctor.

• Bowel changes

Diarrhea, as well as constipation, are common with anxiety. Usually a high-fiber supplement like Metamucil will help regulate your stools.

These are just a few of the more common signs and symptoms of acute and chronic anxiety. No patient will have them all and may have different ones at different times in the course of the disease.

The following are common phobias:

• *Social phobia* is the *fear of situations* in which a person can be watched by others, such as public speaking, or in which the behaviors that arise from the person's feelings might prove embarrassing, such as eating in public. These phobias begin in late childhood or early adolescence.

• *Simple phobia* is the *fear of a situation or specific objects that cause terror*. The condition can begin at any age. Examples are fear of snakes, fear of flying, or fear of enclosed spaces. Some of these phobias are often normal in early childhood, such as fear of the dark.

• *Agoraphobia* is the *fear of being in a public place that has no es cape from crowds*. This is perhaps the most disabling anxiety because victims can become housebound. The illness can begin at any time from late childhood onward.

APPETITE CONTROL

Terry is a 40-year-old, 5 foot 6-inch mother of three who weighs 210 pounds. She has been overweight most of her life and now has been diagnosed with type 2 diabetes (non-insulin dependent diabetes mellitus). She attempts to reduce to her "ideal" weight of 130 pounds. Terry has tried many different types of diets in the past but has never been able to maintain this loss for long. She tells her doctor, "I overeat carbohydrates and I crave them much too much to give them up."

Actually, weight and health do not necessarily go hand in hand. Fitness and health are coupled much closer, and the weight of a person who is really fit may well be much heavier than the doctor's wall chart declares to be healthy.

Appetite control and, more importantly, weight control have been major goals in the lives of most Americans for the greater part of this century. Ever since the mass media has featured advertisements portraying women with hour-glass figures and men with the bodies of Hercules, Americans have been on a quest that few of us have been able to fulfill. Add to this the fact that obesity is a danger and a detriment to health and longevity, and it hasn't taken long for opportunists to create a weight-loss industry that siphons billions of dollars from our pockets each year. And to make matters worse, usually the only weight we lose is the weight of the cash flow out of our pockets.

It hasn't always been that way. Our weight-off mania is a 20th-century phenomenon, spurred on by Madison Avenue, the movies, and insurance companies that invented an arbitrary weight chart to hang on doctors' office walls. Many people are surprised to find out that these charts, which have dictated our "correct" weight for most of this century, were not invented by medical and health researchers but rather by insurance company actuaries, whose interest was not so much in our health but in their companies' profits. Actually, weight and health do not necessarily go hand in hand. Fitness and health are coupled much closer, and the weight of a person who is really fit may well be much heavier than the doctor's wall chart declares to be healthy.

Carbohydrate Cravings and Serotonin

Why does Terry, from the opening story of this chapter, crave carbohydrates? Richard and Judith Wurtman, two researchers for the Massachusetts Institute of Technology, think that low Serotonin levels are involved in eating disturbances. They theorized that overeaters are attempting to self-medicate by loading up on carbohydrates in an attempt to elevate their mood. It works this way: Dietary carbohydrate is metabolized to sugar, the sugar stimulates the pancreas to release insulin, insulin increases brain levels of the amino acid tryptophan, tryptophan is converted into Serotonin, and the Serotonin is then available to regulate mood and produce a sense of well-being. The problem here is that insulin also enhances the storage of fat, so too many carbohydrates can result in a weight gain.

Other researchers have found that premenstrual women and smokers trying to quit also tend to eat more carbohydrates, which seems to lift their mood.

Obesity and the Serotonin Reuptake Inhibitors

By 1980 investigators suspected a link between serotonin and eating disorders. This suspicion was confirmed with the discovery that the Serotonin reuptake inhibitor fluoxetine (Prozac) sometimes produced a side effect of weight loss. Later studies showed that Serotonin-enhancing drugs helped overeaters reduce snacking and lose weight; now the SSRis are being increasingly prescribed to suppress appetite in people who want to lose weight.

Obesity and 5-HTP

Terry wanted to try medication to help her to lose weight but was afraid of the serious side effects she had heard about on the news. She asked her doctor for a more natural alternative. First, he suggested she reconsider her goal of 130 pounds. A 10% loss in body weight was far more realistic and was all she needed to regain her health. Second, her doctor suggested a trial of 5-HTP. He explained how this Serotonin precursor naturally increased Serotonin levels. Now Terry takes 50 mg of 5-HTP before each meal and another 50 mg before bed. She said, "For the first time I feel I am in control of how much I eat." One year later Terry is 40 pounds thinner and there is no sign of her diabetes.

Since drugs that increase Serotonin decrease appetite, it seems logical to suspect that 5-HTP may share these properties. This indeed has been the case.

"I ask people if they have trouble leaving food on their plate, and if they do, I give them 5-HTP. I start with very low doses, like 5 or 10 mg, and with each meal I titrate up and ask the patient to take one additional pill until they can feel themselves not want the food midmeal. When they can feel themselves not want the food midmeal, that's their dose."

Dr. Elisa Lotter is a naturopathic physician in Santa Barbara, California, who often recommends 5-HTP for menopause and weight loss. She says, "I think that part of the eating is self-medication. Part of the excessive exercise is self-medication. And if people are at the homeostatic state that they seek to be at, they can cease extreme behaviors. So, yes, the 5-HTP by increasing the Serotonin level, in reality does control the excess consumption of carbohydrates."

Dr. Lotter remembers a patient who had been on a three month carbohydrate-free diet as part of a program for obsessive eaters. "These people who binge out, they are not bingeing out on carrots, they are not bingeing out on fruits and vegetables, they are bingeing out on carbohydrates. Eating whole loaves of bread. One woman said she had eaten 20,000 calories at one sitting. It is my contention that people who have these extreme eating disorders have physiological low Serotonin levels.

"The 5-HTP really helps. I usually start out with a small dose of 50 mg in the evening, up to 900 mg. Too much too fast and they can get vascular headaches, sinus congestion, and stomach upsets like diarrhea. I start with 50 mg at night for three days and 100 mg at night for another three days."

One study found that 5-HTP can act as an appetite suppressant at low doses (50 to 200 mg), if taken one-half hour before meals. During clinical trials in obese subjects, the intake of 5-HTP caused a voluntary decrease in caloric intake of both carbohydrates and fats, but not of protein. A significant loss of weight occurred, due to a voluntary decrease in caloric intake and not because of a restrictive diet.

An Italian double-blind, crossover study concluded that 5-HTP could be safely used as an obesity treatment. In the study, 20 obese female subjects were given either 5-HTP (8 mg/ kg/ day) or a placebo for five weeks, during which time patients were not prescribed any dietary restrictions. It was found that 5-HTP administration promoted a decrease in appetite and carbohydrate intake that resulted in significant weight loss (approximately 5%) during the period, compared to no significant change in body weight with the placebo controlled subjects.

Dr. Christian Renna is a family practitioner in Texas who specializes in preventative medicine. He uses 5-HTP extensively to treat depression, anxiety, insomnia, and as a weight loss aide. He talks about one of his patients.

James was a successful 45 ear-old insurance broker diagnosed with borderline hypertension and obesity. James's favorite appetizer was Budweiser. James's favorite dessert was Budweiser. Altogether, James consumed about 600 calories a day from beer. He also had difficulty controlling his appetite during the evening meal. Dr. Renna prescribed 15 mg of 5-HTP the first night and that did not prevent James from asking for seconds. He added an additional 15 mg per night. When he reached 60 mg, he was able to stop eating midmeal because he didn't want the food anymore. James said, "I just felt myself lose my appetite in the middle of supper. "

"I ask people if they have trouble leaving food on their plate, and if they do, I give them 5-HTP," says Dr. Renna. "I start with very low doses, like 5 or 10 mg, and with each meal I titrate up and ask the patient to take one additional capsule until they can feel themselves not want the food midmeal. When they can feel themselves not want the food midmeal, that's their dose.

'James lost 20 pounds, which was 10% of his body weight. The downstream effect of having lost this weight was a normalized blood pressure. He was also able to decrease his appetite and consumption of beer.

"I also had a 300-pound patient, and 5-HTP did the same thing for the 300-pound patient that it did for James, the 200-pound patient, although over a much longer period, 15 months.

Now, did the patient lose the 100 pounds because of the 5-HTP? Yes and no. He lost 100 pounds because 5-HTP gave him control of his appetite. Then he used that control to reformulate his diet, and the reformulation of his diet gave him greater energy, and he used the greater energy to institute a program of greater exercise, in this patient's case, walking. And in 15 months, this person lost 100 pounds."

Is this Dr. Renna's typical result with 5-HTP? "The typical result is the ability to gain control over impulsive behavior. The atypical result is to lose over 10% of their body weight. It's very difficult for anyone to lose more than 10% of their body weight. But they can gain all the health benefits of weight reduction with only a 10% loss."

How Much Weight Loss Is Enough?

That is not to say that being fat is good for you or that obesity is not a health threat! Far from it. What we're saying is, forget your weight and get fit! But doesn't getting fit mean losing weight? Not necessarily! It does mean losing some fat, but that does not necessarily mean losing weight. When you get fit, not only may you lose little or no weight, you may even gain a few pounds, depending on where you start out. The reason is that when you get fit, you will gain muscle at the same time that you lose fat, and muscle weighs more than fat, so in the trade-off you may put on a few pounds. But it is a good trade, healthy muscle weight for unhealthy fat weight.

What Is Obesity?

Obesity is surprisingly difficult to define, considering how much we constantly talk about it, fret over it, and detest it. If we compare a person to the statistics on a weight chart and find that he is 5 feet 8 inches tall and weighs 233 pounds, is he obese? The weight chart tells us he should be between 140 and 170 pounds, depending on his bone structure, whether he has a small, medium, or large frame. The chart says he's at least 65 pounds, and maybe even 93 pounds, "overweight." Is he obese?

What if he's a pro football running back without any excess fat? Would you call him "fatty" to his face? Maybe, if you're a linebacker weighing twice that much and just as trim. But the weight chart places him at anywhere from 30% to 60% overweight. Unhealthy? Only according to the weight chart! This guy is heavy but very fit. Much more fit than most of the people who are right on the mark, according to the wall chart!

So if we define obesity as being excessive body fat deposits in a quantity that is detrimental to health, who is obese? The generally agreed upon consensus of doctors and other authorities is that men with more than 25% body fat and women with more than 30% body fat are to be considered obese. Age also enters into the picture and the statistics are a bit more forgiving as we get older.

If we compare a couch potato to the weight chart and he's 5 feet 8 inches tall, small-boned, and weighs in at 170 pounds, is he obese? He might be only 30 pounds overweight, or 20% above what he should be. Is he obese? Unhealthy? Probably! Especially if he's been on the couch long enough to more closely resemble *mashed* potatoes. But according to the weight chart, he's not as dangerously obese as the running back.

To make the problem even more complicated, the *Body Mass Index*, or *BMH*, which is all the rage today and is an attempt to get away from the less flexible doctor's wall chart, will also make our running back look like he's an obese blob and will be more forgiving to Mr. Mashed Potatoes on the couch. Ironically, the blob on the couch can probably buy life insurance easier than the running back who's in tip-top shape.

So how do we define obesity if the wall chart and the BMI don't give us a clue? We don't like any definition of obesity that depends on weight. Obesity should be dependent on excessive body fat and its effect on health. When you have so much excess body fat that it becomes a health risk factor, then you are obese, regardless of your weight. And if you have relatively little body fat on your small, medium, or heavy frame, you're not obese, regardless of your weight.

Some authorities say that if you are even 10% over your designated correct body weight, you've raised your health risk factor. Again, is that fat weight or healthy muscle weight? We'd be more concerned if you were under the average weight and you could pinch up a handful of fat when you grabbed at your gut than if you weighed 30 pounds over the "designated normal" and boasted tight skin over hard abdominal muscle.

Let's try to forget weight, weight charts, and BMI; instead, let's look for a lack of fitness. If you appear to be a mass of fat; if you find yourself weak, easily exhausted, and short of breath when you walk any distance on flat terrain, much less uphill; if you find that your skin hangs heavily away from the muscle that should be beneath it, you are probably obese or well on the way to it.

Experience with 5-HTP here, and especially in Europe, indicates that it has a positive effect on Serotonin, enabling it to restore itself to the quantitiesthat are necessary to reduce our appetite cravings. Thus, 5-HTP makes it easier to decrease our caloric intake.

Maybe the best way to define obesity is to look at its causes. It might surprise you to discover that the obese are basically malnourished! Over nourished, yes, but definitely malnourished.

A properly nourished person is rarely obese! Furthermore, an obese person is under exercised. He or she can never burn off excess storage fat, and because of that, the storage fat keeps adding and adding and adding up. So perhaps obesity is a lifestyle problem. Maybe we should define obesity as a disease that develops out of a lifestyle that is lacking in exercise, coupled with malnourishment.

There are a few rare causes of obesity that must be differentiated from lifestyle causes, another reason why a complete physical examination should be carried out before considering any form of therapy and exercise or any other treatment of obesity. These other possible etiologies of obesity include hypothyroidism, Cushing's syndrome, depression, and certain rare neurological pathologies that can lead to overeating. Occasionally, medications such as steroids and certain antidepressants can cause excessive weight gain. In these cases, treatment should be aimed at the etiologic condition rather than at the weight gain they have caused. Your physician should be able to make an accurate diagnosis and treat the underlying problem, or else refer you to the proper specialist. Appetite suppressants would seldom if ever be indicated in these treatments unless they have been long-standing and eating habits need to be markedly altered.

But what are the symptoms and signs of this disease called obesity? If we rule out weight and overweight as criteria, then perhaps the percentage of fat should be our guide. Although the percentage of internal body fat does increase with increased weight, approximately 50% of all body fat is deposited in and just under the skin. This makes for a simple and inexpensive, as well as a fairly accurate, way to gauge body fat percentages by the skinfold measurement, which works nearly as well as most high tech electronic resistance methods or the awkward water emersion. This skinfold method will measure your total percentage of body fat to within 3% to 4% of accuracy in the hands of an experienced appraiser, and when one considers all the variables that can creep into the more high tech methods, it is probably just as accurate in evaluating obesity.

In the skinfold method, a caliper is used to measure the thickness of pinched-up skinfolds in specific areas of the body. These readings are then applied to a chart with a scale of the percentage of your body mass that is attributable to fat. In some medical offices as well as in some health clubs you might find a *Bioelectric Impedance Analyzer*, a device that is able to measure the difference in resistance between the flow of electricity through muscle and through fat and thus determine with fair accuracy the percentage of fat in the body. These machines are becoming more common in physician's offices. Either method is accurate enough for diagnosing obesity.

So if we define obesity as being excessive body fat deposits in a quantity that is detrimental to health, who is obese? The generally agreed-upon consensus of doctors and other authorities is that men with more than 25% body fat and women with more than 30% body fat are to be considered obese. Age also enters into the picture and the statistics are a bit more forgiving as we get older.

Remember, these obesity and excess fat percentage risks are also affected by other factors. If you are under great stress, smoke cigarettes, eat foods that are poor in nutritional value, have high blood triglycerides and high cholesterol, have high blood pressure, are diabetic, do not exercise regularly in a vig orous aerobic program, and/or have a family history of heart disease, you may be pushed into a high risk category even though your body fat is only in the low to moderate range.

A low percentage of body fat is no guaranteed indicator- of health status. It is only one risk factor among many. There are thin people of relatively poor health and relatively fat people in extremely good health. True, a thin person who is fit has a much better chance of being in good health than a more portly person, but not all thin people are fit and not all heavy folks are unfit.

So, having defined *obesity* as a "*disease* determined by the *quantity of body fat* sufficient to become a *health risk*, usually in the range of 25% *in men* and 30% *in women*," let's get on with the essence of this topic.

How Does Obesity Kill?

Obesity kills by predisposing you to one or more terminal illnesses. Obese people are twice as likely to die prematurely as are non-obese individuals. Obesity is significantly linked to diabetes, heart disease, hypertension, stroke, and cancers of the colon, rectum, prostate, breast, gallbladder, uterus, cervix, and ovaries, to name a few. Obesity is also associated with nonfatal, but often debilitating, chronic health problems such as gallbladder disease and gallstones, osteoarthritis, gout, pulmonary problems, and sleep apnea. Let's take a closer look.

Hypertension

Even in younger obese patients between the ages of 20 and 40, the prevalence of hypertension is 6 to 10 times greater than in persons of normal weight. Hypertension can eventually lead to stroke, heart attack or failure, kidney failure, detached retina and blindness, aneurism and/or arterial rupture, and other terminal conditions. The younger you are when you begin developing hypertension, the greater the chance you have of developing one or more of these potentially terminal problems.

Diabetes

Even mild to moderate obesity can increase the risk of developing non-insulin dependent diabetes mellitus by a multiple of ten. This is especially so if you carry a large portion of your excess storage fat in the abdominal area of your torso. Fatty tissue tends to increase your chance of developing non-insulin dependent diabetes mellitus in two ways: first, by increasing the body's demand for insulin, causing the pancreas to have difficulty in keeping up with the demand; and second, by increasing resistance to insulin by the cells of the body. Since the *adipose*, or fatty, tissue is resistant to the insulin, it remains in storage rather than being burned off as energy. Furthermore, ingested fats are more likely to be deposited into storage, creating a vicious cycle. Reducing the percentage of body fat by cutting calories and increasing exercise, combined with cultivating well-balanced nutritional habits, can reverse this detrimental cycle and push diabetes into remission.

Diabetes increases your chances of developing renal failure; heart disease; stroke; blindness; circulatory problems, which can lead to gangrene and the amputation of limbs or even death; chronic skin ulcerations, which can lead to lethal infections; and severe neurological problems.

Cardiovascular Diseases

Obesity, cardiac disease, and death go hand in hand, independent of all other risk factors. In other words, regardless of all other lifestyle risk factors such as smoking, chemical abuse, and stresses that may or may not be part of your daily life, obesity alone can bring on heart disease and mortality. Obesity is usually accompanied by elevated *cholesterol* levels, especially the *low density lipids (WL) cholesterol*, otherwise known as *bad cholesterol*.

LDL cholesterol is directly related to coronary artery disease, coronary occlusion, and death from cardiac arrest. The incidence of *congestive heart failure (CHF)* and its morbidity and mortality are also closely related to obesity. Elevated blood pressure usually accompanies obesity, along with a taxing of the heart muscle, which has to circulate blood through hundreds of miles of extra venules, capillaries, and arterioles that run throughout the mass of adipose tissue. This weakens the heart muscle until it becomes an inefficient pump, and a dam forms causing fluid to build up in the lungs, virtually drowning the individual in his or her own fluids.

Cancer

Obesity in men is closely connected to the incidence of numerous cancers, which collectively cost millions of lives each year. Colorectal cancer is two to three times greater in obese men than in their less corpulent brethren. Prostate cancer is also two to three times more likely to attack the obese. Obese women also have a much greater chance of developing cancers of the breast, gallbladder, uterus, cervix, and ovaries, which raises their mortality rates dramatically over women of slimmer build. In cultures where obesity is not nearly as prevalent as in the United States, the incidence of these dreaded diseases is much lower.

Stroke

The hypertension and the hypercholesterolemia that occur in conjunction with obesity both increase the incidence of strokes in fat folks. The brain uses more oxygen than any organ of the body and depends on an unimpeded flow of oxygenated blood. When that flow is interrupted, either because a blood vessel ruptures under high blood pressure or because an artery or arteriole becomes clogged from the buildup of cholesterol, the brain tissue that the blood flow nourishes will quickly die. The tragic result is a stroke whose damage is all too frequently permanent; severe disability or death will usually follow.

Chronic Diseases

Not all diseases that trouble the obese are potentially terminal, but, nonetheless, they may cost the patient dearly in terms of physical and financial suffering, drastically diminishing his or her quality of life.

Menstruation and Pregnancy

Obese women are far more likely to have menstrual irregularities and difficulties in achieving conception than women of normal weight. If pregnancy is accomplished, the incidence of miscarriage, diabetes, toxemia, and hypertension is much more likely to complicate the gestation period.

Both men and women who are obese tend to court a higher risk of gallstones and gallbladder disease, including gallbladder cancer. These patients suffer from severe pain, digestive disorders, and eventually surgical intervention. Gallbladder disease can be a serious complication during pregnancy for obese women.

Sleep Apnea

Sleep apnea is a problem closely connected with obesity. It manifests in long periods during which the breath stops due to a mechanical obstruction of the airway; this is caused by enlarged and redundant adipose tissue surrounding the air passage. There have been a few cases of death due to sleep apnea, but more often it results in such a poor quality of sleep that the individual cannot work efficiently during the day and frequently falls asleep at work or even while driving.

Absenteeism among obese people is much greater than among other workers and students.

If you are considered overweight according to the standard height and weight measurements on a chart, your size may be due to healthy muscle and organ tissue. If, on the other hand, you are heavy due to a high percentage of body fat, which in our culture is all too often the case, then you may be in serious danger of morbid or mortal illness, one of which is sleep apnea. If you are fat but not yet obese, you probably will be obese in the not-too-distant future unless you do some thing to turn yourself around now! The human body is not a status quo object, it either deteriorates or it improves. If you don't do something actively to make it improve, we guarantee that you will further deteriorate.

What Is the Role of 5-HTP
in My Weight Loss and Control Program?

Experience with 5-HTP here, and especially in Europe, indicates that it has qualities that are necessary to reduce our appetite cravings. Thus, 5-HTP makes it easier to decrease our caloric intake. However, no pill or capsule, prescription or over-the counter supplement, no matter how powerful or effective, can take off your excessive fat or maintain your weight all by itself. There is no magic in 5-HTP or in any other weight-loss medication or device. You must make some basic changes in your lifestyle in order to accomplish your goal of fitness.

There is a very simple formula for weight gain and loss, and any medication, supplement, device, salve, potion, or fitness program must adhere to this simple formula. It is simply this: "If you take in more calories than you burn off in energy, then you will gain excess fat; if you take in fewer calories than you burn off in energy, then you will burn off your excess fat."

Let's repeat that statement: "If you take in more calories than you bum off in energy, then you will gain excess fat; if you take in fewer calories than you bum off in energy, then you will bum off your excess fat." There is no way around this basic fact. If you want to get rid of your excessive fat baggage, then you have to burn off more calories in the form of work and exercise than you eat. And, no, sitting on your couch watching TV is not considered exercise or work and neither is chewing on snacks. Yet this is the favorite pastime of all too many Americans, and, sadly, most kids as well. America has never been more health conscious than at present, and Americans have never been fatter than we are now, either. Being conscious of fitness is not enough, you have to do something about it.

Yes, taking 5-HTP is doing something about it. It will make cutting your caloric intake easier, but by itself it won't be enough. You must make two major changes in your lifestyle. One, you have to eat a more nutritious diet, meaning you need to eat balanced meals with low fat and high fiber content; and two, you have to get rid of your excess fat by going out to exercise. Now, that's not nearly as bad as it may sound at first. You'll notice that we didn't say go on a diet. We said that you need to eat more nutritiously. If you eat nutritiously, you can cut your calories considerably without reducing the quantity of food you eat. This is because fat has more than twice the calories that carbohydrates and protein have, and fiber has virtually no caloric value.

And the exercise program need not be threatening, either. Simple brisk walking will burn off calories and tone and build muscles that you thought you'd never see again.

Go out and take that first walk of your new lifestyle right now, and repeat it every day from now on, lengthening it and picking up speed as you enjoy new health and strength and fitness.

SLEEP DISORDERS

Thomas has been having trouble sleeping for the past five years, but since his retirement last year at age 65 the situation has gotten worse. It takes more than an hour for Tom to fall asleep at night, and he frequently awakens in the middle of the night and is unable to fall sleep again. Tom has tried over-the-counter sleeping aids and finally asked his physician for "sleeping pills."

Virtually everyone has and will again encounter sleep problems at various times in their lives. Sleep problems are with us from infancy to the grave, but for most of us they are transient and intermittent. Nevertheless, for many people they are a serious and constant plague.

Over 70 million Americans suffer from a sleep problem, nearly one-third of our population, and for nearly 60% of these people, sleep difficulties are a serious chronic disorder. The most common sleep problem is insomnia, the inability to fall asleep or to stay asleep long enough to get a good and healthful night's rest. Furthermore, like Thomas, well over half of all Americans aged 65 and older have a sleep problem.

The prevalence of sleep disorders appears to increase with advancing age, and as Americans grow older an estimated 80 million will suffer a chronic and serious sleep problem by the year 2015. Sleep disorders cost Americans well over an estimated $15 billion addition to our national health care bill. And it's not just the aged who are suffering from chronic loss of sleep; about 25% of American children between the ages of one and five have a serious sleep disturbance that disrupts their rest, while also causing sleep loss and anxiety for their parents.

Sleep is an essential component of human behavior. Nearly a third of the life of a normal adult is spent sleeping. Normal sleep is divided into rapid eye movement (REM) and non-REM sleep. REM sleep is characterized by a low amplitude pattern in the EEG, or electroencephalogram, with an associated loss of muscle tone and the presence of rapid eye movements. Non REM sleep, on the other hand, is characterized by sleep spindles and slow wave activity in the EEG. This regulation of sleep reflects basic brain mechanisms that provide for the organization of both behavioral and physiological processes.

Tryptophan and Sleep

Tryptophan was a commonly used over-the-counter sleep-inducing agent that enjoyed great success in the treatment of insomnia. Although tryptophan is the precursor to both Serotonin, the neurohormone that mediates sleep, and melatonin, the neurohormone involved in the sleep-wake cycle, tryptophan appears _ to have sleep-enhancing properties unique to itself. Perhaps for this reason, many practitioners have found tryptophan superior to 5-HTP for inducing deep sleep in those not troubled by depression. However, 5-HTP is effective as well, and it is not uncommon to take both tryptophan and 5-HTP together.

The amount of tryptophan used for insomnia ranges from 500 to 3,000 mg per day. Presently, it is only available by prescription.

Serotonin and Sleep

As you will remember from the first chapter, Serotonin itself cannot cross the blood-brain barrier. The Serotonin used in the brain must be manufactured there from tryptophan, an amino acid that *can* cross the blood-brain barrier. However, it has been estimated that only 1% of the tryptophan we ingest in our diets ever reaches the brain.

Among its many neurotransmitter duties, Serotonin works to modulate the sleep state. When Serotonin levels drop, one of the results is insomnia. Serotonin is one of three monoamines found in the brain. The others are dopamine and noradrenalin, formed from the amino acid tyrosine. These neurotransmitters promote over-arousal, tension, anxiety, and sleep disturbances. Serotonin offsets the effects of these chemicals. When you eat a high protein meal, brain levels of tyrosine rise and more of these neurotransmitters are manufactured than Serotonin. When you eat a high carbohydrate meal, the insulin secreted by the pancreas clears the other competing amino acids out of the blood and into cells. In other words, carbohydrates work to get tryptophan into the brain.

Over 70 million Americans suffer from a sleep problem, nearly one-third of our population, and for nearly 60% of these people, sleep difficulties are a serious chronic disorder. The most common sleep problem is insomnia, the inability to fall asleep or to stay asleep long enough to get a good and healthful night's rest.

Melatonin

Melatonin is the neurohormone responsible for regulation of the sleep-wake cycle. It is produced from Serotonin in the Pineal gland, especially at night. When light enters the eye, melatonin production is suppressed. Melatonin is used by many travelers to eliminate jet lag.

Since melatonin is produced from Serotonin, taking supplements of 5-HTP also raises your melatonin levels. When a group of researchers gave 5-HTP to sheep, it increased their serum melatonin levels more than sevenfold within two hours. It may be that some of the benefits enjoyed for 5-HTP are more the result of higher melatonin levels than of higher Serotonin levels.

Serotonin is also a growth hormone releaser. Growth hormone is usually secreted only during deep sleep and is crucial for growth, repair, and maintenance of the immune system. One of the effects of low Serotonin levels is poor growth hormone secretion, which is commonly seen in the elderly, the obese, or those with fibromyalgia.

5-HTP and Sleep

The direct precursor to Serotonin, the neurotransmitter involved in sleep, is 5-HTP. Since 5-HTP is known for its ability to relieve depression and anxiety, it is the perfect choice of a sleep agent in those who have insomnia due to worry, depression, or anxiety. Let us again look at the case of Thomas, our retiree with insomnia.

Thomas's doctor surprised him by not wanting to give him sleeping pills. He suspected that part of Thomas' problem was anxiety due to his unwanted retirement. He also knew that Thomas had had very poor eating habits for most of his life and was probably not getting all the nutrients his body needed to slip easily into sleep. He sent Thomas home with instructions to include a multimineral and vitamin supplement at each meal and to take 100 mg of 5-HTP one hour before bed time. Within a week of starting this program, Thomas was able to sleep through the night.

One of the great benefits of 5-HTP is its lack of side effects. The main side effects of 5-HTP are gastrointestinal; nausea, diarrhea, and abdominal pain. These problems can usually be avoided by starting on a low dose of 25 to 50 mg before bedtime. Some people may have to start as low as 5 to 10 mg. Once the body has adjusted to this amount, it can be slowly increased until jt reaches a therapeutic dose. Sleeping pills, on the other hand, often leave people with a hung-over feeling the next morning.

Karen had chronic insomnia for years. She worked for a software company in a job that required accurate information management. She was taking double the normal dose of Dalmane, a benzodiazepine used for insomnia. As a side effect, it caused a mild impairment in memory and mental function that made Karen's job more difficult. She asked her doctor if a replacement was possible. Karen and her doctor attempted to wean her off of Dalmane and onto 5-HTP. She started to take the 5-HTP and in three months she was able to cut the dose of Dalmane in half. After nine months, she was totally off Dalmane and now takes 400 mg of 5-HTP each night.

Karen was able to substitute a heavy sleep medication for one with no side effects.

Research in France found that 100 mg of 5-HTP resulted in significant improvement in the sleep of people described as "mildly insomniac." A Norwegian scientist examining sleep patterns in cats found that 5-HTP had effects on sleep that were similar to those produced by tryptophan.

What Is Insomnia?

Insomnia is the difficulty of either initiating sleep and/or maintaining sleep of an adequate quality and quantity to provide sufficient rest in order to function during waking hours. Although insomnia is a term often misused to indicate any and all types of sleep loss, it is not a disorder at all but rather a symptom of other disorders.

Sleep Disturbance in Cancer Patients

Cancer patients are at great risk for developing insomnia and disorders of the sleep cycle. Insomnia is the most common sleep disturbance in this population and is usually secondary to physical and/or psychological factors related to the cancer and/or its treatment. Anxiety and depression are common psychological responses to the diagnosis of cancer, cancer treatment, and hospitalization, and the anxiety and depression are often accompanied by insomnia. Sleep disturbances may be exacerbated by syndromes associated with steroid production, steroid treatment, and by symptoms associated with tumor invasion, such as draining lesions, gastrointestinal and genitourinary pain, fever, cough, dyspnea, itching, and fatigue. Medications, including vitamins, corticosteroids, neuroleptics for nausea and vomiting, as well as other treatment factors can negatively impact sleep patterns.

Hospitalized patients are likely to experience frequent interruptions of sleep due to treatment schedules, hospital routines, and roommates, which singularly or collectively alter the sleep-wake schedule. Other factors influencing sleep-wake schedules in the hospital setting include age, noise, temperature, comfort, pain, and anxiety.

One of the great benefits of 5-HTP is its lack of side effects. The main side effects of 5-HTP are gastrointestinal nausea, diarrhea, and abdominal pain. These problems can usually be avoided by starting on a low dose of 25 to 50 mg before bedtime. Some people may have to start as low as 5 to 10 mg. Once the body has adjusted to this amount, it can be slowly increased until it reaches a therapeutic dose. Sleeping pills, on the other hand, often leave people with a hungover feeling the next morning.

Supplemental 5-HTP has been used quite extensively in

Europe for the relief of cancer pain and has been noted to help induce sleep, whether from its pain-relieving features, its Serotonin effect, or both. Because it will most likely be taken with other cancer-treating drugs, you should always discuss its use with your doctor.

Sleepwalking (Somnambulism)

Sleepwalking, or somnambulism, is a series of complex behaviors that are initiated during slow wave sleep and that result in actual walking and activity during sleep. Symptoms include walking and moving about, which occur while a person is still sleeping. The onset typically occurs in prepubertal children. Characteristics of sleepwalking include: difficulty in arousing the patient during a somnambulistic episode and amnesia following an episode; these episodes typically occur early in the first third of the sleep period; monitoring demonstrates the onset of an episode during stage 3 or 4 sleep; other medical and psychiatric disorders can be present but do not necessarily account for the symptoms; and the ambulation is not due to other sleep disorders, such as sleep terrors.

In some people, sleepwalking occurs less than once per month and does not result in harm to either the sleepwalker or others, while other people experience episodes more than once a month, but not nightly, and the activity does not harm anyone. However, in the most severe form of sleepwalking, the episodes occur almost nightly and can result in physical injury. Further more, the sleepwalker may feel embarrassment, shame, guilt, anxiety, and confusion when told about his sleepwalking behavior. If the problem becomes so severe that the sleepwalker exits the house or is having frequent episodes and injuries are occurring, it is time to seek professional help.

Very often sleepwalking is triggered by overwork, worry,

anxiety, and stress. These are all states that can be alleviated by 5-HTP. A person prone to sleepwalking might be well advised to take 5-HTP along with him on any stressful business trips and use it as a preventative measure. Again, keep in mind that 5-HTP should not be combined with prescription medications except on the advice of a health care professional.

Sleep Bruxism

Sleep bruxism is characterized by a grinding or clenching of the teeth during sleep. Bruxism may cause abnormal wear of the teeth and jaw muscle discomfort that can be quite painful. It sounds about as pleasant as fingernails on a chalkboard and is guaranteed to drive your bed partner nuts. Some episodes occur less than nightly, with no evidence of dental injury or impairment of psychosocial functioning. Other people experience nightly episodes, with evidence of mild impairment of psychosocial functioning and mild dental damage, and yet others have nightly episodes with evidence of more severe dental injury and temporomandibular joint and jaw disorders.

Before you invest large amounts of money in jaw splints, begin a two-week trial of 5-HTP to see if it helps. Since 5-HTP is an excellent stress-reducer, it may give you a deeper sleep, free of tension.

Sleep and the Elderly

Sleep of the elderly person differs from that of a younger person in several ways:

1. The older adult experiences numerous brief arousals during the night. In men, this is partly due to the need to evacuate the bladder, especially if the person has benign prostatic hypertrophy (BPH), or enlargement of the prostate gland.

2. With age, there is a loss of the deepest levels of non-REM sleep, stages 3 and 4 deep sleep.

3. There is more daytime napping among the elderly, which probably causes nighttime sleep to be less deep, as was noted in #2. This can create a cycle of poor quality sleep at night, requiring more sleep during the day, leading to more poor quality sleep at night. This type of insomnia might well be helped by taking 5-HTP, which might deepen the nighttime sleep and interrupt the cycle of poor nighttime sleep and a daytime need for napping.

4. The elderly experience less of a drop in body temperature during sleep, probably due to the fact that stages 3 and 4 sleep are not as deep. Temperature and metabolism both normally become lower during these stages.

5. The elderly tend toward having earlier bedtimes and also earlier wake-ups.

6. The elderly have a greater tendency to suffer from sleep apnea, or the cessation of breathing during sleep, which causes brief arousals in order to begin breathing again; this prevents sleep from getting as deep as it should. Apnea is more common in men than in women.

7. The elderly have an increased incidence of myoclonic activity, or muscular jerking and twitching, which often briefly awakens them.

8. The elderly have more frequent and more serious medical problems, such as heart failure, breathing problems, gastric reflux, and chronic pain from arthritis and other illnesses, which keep them from getting quality sleep. Since 5-HTP has some pain-reducing properties, as well as sleepinducing benefits, it might work well in these situations.

9. Psychiatric disorders in the elderly commonly impair their sleep, as do dementia and senility. There is often an increase in agitation and disorientation among the elderly at night; more often, this occurs in the demented elderly patient. Supplemental 5-HTP might help to settle this type of nighttime agitation by deepening sleep.

10. Poor sleep habits, such as an irregular sleep schedule; evening nicotine, caffeine, or alcohol; adverse conditioning caused by spending too much time in bed; and a poor sleeping environment can lead to impaired sleep. These conditions are more likely to occur among the elderly.

The Stages of Sleep

The Normal Sleep Stages

• In stage 0 sleep you are still awake, but your bodily activity slows down and your muscle tension decreases. You are at borderline wakefulness, drowsy, and your muscles begin to relax, your mind relaxes and awareness dulls; your heart rate, blood pressure, and body temperature begin to diminish.

• In stage 1 sleep, your eyes roll slowly upward and you feel sleepy; you are indeed in a light sleep, easily awakened by interfering thoughts, sounds, or stimulation. Your body movements are markedly slowed and your temperature and heart rate slow further, breathing becomes slow and regular, and you may have hypnotic hallucinations and dream activity while falling to sleep.

Supplemental 5-HTP has been used quite extensively in Europe for the relief of cancer pain and has been noted to help induce sleep, whether from its pain-relieving features, its serotonin effect, or both.

• In stage 2 sleep, eye movements slow and snoring may take place. Awakening is still relatively easy. If your eyes open in this stage, they will be non-seeing. You may have some thought fragments, but memory processes diminish rapidly and dreams may be vaguely remembered if you are awakened. Heart rate, blood pressure, and temperature continue to diminish, but breathing, though regular, may encounter more airway resistance as muscles relax. Snoring may increase.

• In stage 3 sleep, eyes move only on rare occasions and deep sleep ensues, with only loud sounds causing reawakening. Dreaming takes place, but memory is very sketchy. Metabolic rate is slowed, as are all other bodily functions except for the increased secretion of certain hormones, including growth hormone, probably for the restoration of body tissues.

• In stage 4 sleep, there is occasional body movement, the eyes are quiet, you are in a state of deepest sleep, and it is most difficult to awaken. There is virtually no recall of dreams, and thought processes are minimal. Bodily functions continue to slow.

In the fourth stage of sleep is the rapid eye movement (REM) stagewhere the major muscles are virtually paralyzed, although facial muscles, fingers, and toes twitch. Snoring tends to cease. Awakening is difficult, and outside or potentially disturbing sounds are usually incorporated into dreams to protect you from awakening. Dream recall is best in this stage, up to 80%. This stage of dreaming may be involved with subconscious conflict resolution. Bodily functions are slightly increased over the previous stages.

HOSTILITY AND AGGRESSION

Chuck has always had a short temper. He was known as a bully in school and has had trouble keeping girlfriends. He has no patience when caught in traffic and often swears and curses at other drivers. After the death of his father, Chuck became very depressed over the quality of his life. His family doctor feels he should take an antidepressant, but Chuck feels very uneasy about taking drugs.

Hostility and aggressive behavior are actually symptoms or reactions to the emotion we know as anger. We've all experienced anger as either a fleeting annoyance or full-fledged rage. Like anxiety or occasional depression and sadness, anger is a completely normal, usually healthy, human emotion. When it gets out of control and turns destructive, however, it can lead to problems at work, in your personal relationships, in your dealings with strangers, and in everyday activities. You may find yourself at the mercy of an unpredictable and powerful emotion.

Anger is an emotion varying in intensity from mild irritation to intense fury and rage. Like any other emotion, it is accompanied by physiological and biological changes: Your heart rate and blood pressure go up, as does the blood level of the hormones adrenaline and noradrenalin, or norepinephrine, the "fight or flight" neurotransmitters.

Expressing Anger

The instinctive, natural way to express anger is to respond aggressively or with hostility. Anger is a natural response to threats and elicits powerful aggressive feelings and behaviors that allow us to defend ourselves when attacked. A certain degree of anger is necessary to our survival. However, it is not normal for us to lash out at every person or object that irritates or annoys us. Our anger has to be tempered to be socially acceptable, and laws, social norms, and common sense place limits on our anger and on our defensive and aggressive behavior. We use both conscious and unconscious processes to deal with our angry feelings.

Expressing angry feelings in an assertive, nonaggressive manner is the healthiest way to defuse anger. You have to learn how to make clear what your needs are and how to get them satisfied without threatening or hurting others. This needn't mean acting pushy or demanding; it means being respectful of yourself and others.

Anger can also be suppressed, converted, or redirected. This happens when you hold in your anger, stop thinking about it, and focus on something positive. You suppress your anger and convert it into more constructive behavior. The danger of this type of response is that if it isn't allowed outward expression, your anger can turn inward on yourself, leading to serious frustration and self-depreciation. Anger turned inward may cause elevation of blood pressure, further anger, and/or depression.

Serotonin and Hostility

It is clinically significant that a deficit of Serotonin is central to the development of depression, agitation, sleep disorders, obesity, and addiction. For this reason, the pharmaceutical control of brain Serotonin levels is the mechanism of action of the two commonly prescribed classes of drugs used in the treatment of depression. Prozac is an example of a selective

Serotonin reuptake inhibitor (SSRI) that prevents the "presynaptic" nerve from reabsorbing Serotonin that it has previously secreted. By inhibiting this normal process, Prozac causes an increase in brain Serotonin levels and an antidepressant effect. Another class of antidepressant drugs, the monoamine oxidase (MAO) inhibitors, cause an increase in Serotonin levels by preventing its degradation. Conversely, the experimental depletion of Serotonin in animals by eliminating tryptophan from the diet causes an increase in aggressiveness.

A 1992 study led by Dr. Gerdi Weidner, a psychologist at the State University of New York at Stony Brook, followed the progress of 233 families in Portland, Oregon. Those who switched to a diet low in fat and high in complex carbohydrates reduced their cholesterol and experienced less depression and aggressive hostility. The researchers were not clear why a low-fat diet had such an effect, but they speculated that the lower protein levels associated with low-fat diets may be responsible.

Researchers at Vanderbilt University conducted a study that investigated the relationship between increased Serotonin receptor sensitivity and human aggression. They conclude that in those with pre-existing aggressive traits, acute drops in central Serotonin can cause increased subjective and objective aggression, while rises can have the opposite effect. In the group with low aggression, the drops in Serotonin had no effect. This suggests that the primary effect of Serotonin levels may be on impulsivity, possibly mediated by Serotonin-1a receptors, expressing underlying aggressive traits. Other reports had also found that lowering tryptophan levels causes mood changes in certain people. It appears that Serotonin is involved with the "control" of aggression.

Anger and Depression

Since anger frequently has a depressive component, and often sleep deprivation accompanies depression, 5-HTP would probably have a beneficial effect in many cases of prolonged anger. However, there is no evidence that 5-HTP has any effect on the few cases of genetically induced chronic anger and aggression because, in most of those cases, there would usually be an abundance of the precursor to Serotonin at most times.

Chuck went to see a psychiatrist, who recognized that Chuck not only was depressed but had trouble controlling his impulsive behavior. The psychiatrist recommended that Chuck try 5-HTP for his depression. After two months of therapy, not only has the depression over his f ther's death lifted, he now finds his temper much easier to control.

A 1992 study led by Dr. Gerdi Weidner, a psychologist at the State University of New York at Stony Brook, followed the progress of 233 families in Portland, Oregon. Those who switched to a diet low in fat and high in complex carbohydrates reduced their cholesterol and experienced less depression and aggressive hostility. The researchers were not clear why a low-fat diet had such an effect, but they speculated that the lower protein levels associated with low-fat diets may be responsible.

Unexpressed anger can lead to pathological expressions of anger, such as passive-aggressive behavior-getting back at people indirectly, without telling them why, rather than confronting them head-on-or creating a personality that seems perpetually cynical and hostile. Such people are constantly putting others down, criticizing everything, and making cynical comments; they haven't learned how to constructively express their anger and they aren't likely to have many close or successful relationships.

Alternatively, you can calm yourself down, meaning not just control your outward behavior but also control your internal responses, taking steps to lower your heart rate, relax, and let the angry feelings subside. Properly managing anger will reduce the intensity of both your emotional feelings and the physiological arousal that anger causes. You can't completely get rid of, or avoid, the people or things that enrage you, nor can you change them, but you can learn to control your reactions. There are psychological tests that measure the intensity of angry feelings and just how prone to anger you are and how well you handle it; but chances are, if you do have a problem with anger, you already know it. If you constantly find yourself acting in ways that seem out of control and frightening when dealing with others, you might need help with this turbulent emotion.

Some People Are More Angry Than Others

Some people are more hostile than others and get angry more easily and more intensely than the average person; some don't show their anger in loud, spectacular ways but are chronically irritable and grumpy. The fact is, easily angered people don't always curse and throw things; sometimes they withdraw socially, sulk, or get physically ill. Easily angered people generally have a low tolerance for frustration, feeling that they shouldn't have to be subjected to obstacles, inconvenience, or annoyance. They can't take things in stride, and they're particularly infuriated if the situation seems somehow unjust, such as having to wait for something or being criticized for a mistake.

It is clinically significant that a deficit of Serotonin is central to the development of depression, agitation, sleep disorders, obesity, and addiction. For this reason, the pharmaceutical control of brain serotonin levels is the mechanism of action of the two commonly prescribed classes of drugs used in the treatment of depression.

One cause for this "short fuse" type of personality may be genetic or physiological. There is evidence that some people are born irritable and easily angered, and that signs are present from a very early age. Another factor may be environmental, for anger is often regarded as a negative emotion; frequently, we are taught that it's all right to express anxiety, depression, or other emotions but not to express anger. As a result, some of us never learn how to handle anger or channel it constructively. And family background plays an important role since, typically, people who are easily angered come from families that are disruptive, chaotic, and not skilled at emotional communication.

People who overtly express their anger in a very hostile way use the theory "letting it out is healthy" as a license to hurt others. But researchers have found that blasting others with anger actually escalates anger and aggression and does nothing to help you or the person you're angry with resolve the conflict. In fact, the resentment that is raised usually makes the conflict worse and makes mediation and resolution much more difficult.

People who overtly express their anger in a very hostile way use the theory "letting it out is healthy" as a license to hurt others. But researchers have found that blasting others with anger actually escalates anger and aggression and does nothing to help you or the person you're angry with resolve the conflict. In fact, the resentment that is raised usually makes the conflict worse and makes mediation and resolution much more difficult.

Keeping Anger at Bay

Relax! Simple relaxation tools such as deep breathing and soothing imagery can help calm down angry feelings. There are books and courses that can teach you relaxation techniques, and once you learn them you can call upon them in any situation. Breathe deeply, from your diaphragm; breath ing from your chest won't relax you. Slowly repeat a calming word or phrase such as "Relax!" "Ease off!" "Cool down!" "Mellow!" Repeat it to yourself while breathing deeply. Use imagery to visualize a relaxing experience. Non-strenuous, slow, yoga-like exercises can relax your muscles and make you feel much calmer. Even the old trick of counting to ten can make a big difference between flying off the handle and tactfully resolving a conflict.

Problem Solving

Usually, unless we're among those hotheads we've just described, our anger and frustration are caused by very real and inescapable problems. Most mild anger is not misplaced, and often it's a healthy, natural response to everyday problems. It only adds to our frustration to find out that every problem doesn't have a satisfactory solution. The best attitude we can maintain in such a situation is to focus on how to best handle and face the problem. People who cope usually have the attitude "Make the best of the situation" or "Make lemonade out of the lemons!" When a problem arises, resolve to give it your best effort at solution, but also promise not to punish yourself if an answer doesn't present itself right away. If you can approach any problem with your best intentions and efforts and make a serious attempt to face it, you'll be much less likely to lose patience and end up in angry frustration.

Rational Communications

Angry people tend to jump to wild and irrational conclusions. If you are in a heated discussion, slow down and think through your responses. Don't say the first thing that comes to mind; think carefully about what you want to say and listen carefully to what others are saying. Taking your time before answering is much better strategy than flying off the handle and screaming absurdities. Look for what is underlying the anger and see what you can do to defuse it.

Humor

Humor can defuse rage by creating a more balanced perspective. Humor can always be relied on to help un-knot a tense situation. Think of people who have a non-offensive sense of humor and you will find that they cope well with angering situations, usually solve problems satisfactorily, and take life in stride. However, there are two cautions regarding the use of humor. First, don't try to just "laugh off your problems," but in stead use humor to help yourself face them more realistically and constructively. Second, don't give in to harsh, sarcastic humor, which is really just another unhealthy expression of anger and is often the cruelest form of aggression and hostility. Humor is really a refusal to take yourself too seriously.

You Have Behavior Choices

Aggression. Aggressive anger can be expressed either physically, emotionally, or psychologically and the end result is usually that someone else gets hurt. Hitting, kicking, harassment, or using put-downs or threats solve nothing. Your personal satisfaction is usually short-lived and the resultant remorse is not easily forgotten.

Passive aggression . Passive-aggressive anger is repressed by internalizing it and denying that it exists. Internalization of anger may lead to both physical and psychological disorders if it is too frequently used..

Assertiveness. Anger that is resolved into assertiveness is expressed in a nonthreatening manner and does not hurt you, other people, or even property. Acknowledging your feelings and deciding how to best deal with an angering situation is the least frustrating and most satisfactory method of coping. Realize there is no such thing as bad anger or good anger; there are only good and bad choices as to how you deal with your anger.

Causes of Anger

Researchers have found that the most common causes of anger are arguments with family members (25%), conflicts at work (22%), and legal problems (8%). Financial problems, as a category, are also anger-provoking, as is dealing with merchants and businesses. Arguments with teenage children, divorces, and mortgage foreclosures are situations that particularly inflame anger. Anger at bad news that is beyond your control is especially damaging to your health and psyche.

Among the physical dangers produced by anger are heart and cardiovascular disease. A study involving 1,300 older men with a mean age of 62 who were followed over a seven-year period found that men with the highest levels of anger were three times more likely to develop heart disease than men with the lowest levels of anger. The research, led by Dr. Ichiro Kawachi, assistant professor of health and social behavior at the Harvard School of Public Health, and published in the November 1, 1996, AHA journal *Circulation*, also found that the men who scored highest for anger on a personality test were heavier, more likely to be smokers, and more likely to ingest at least two alcoholic drinks a day.

A study at Union Memorial Hospital and Loyola College of Maryland in Baltimore interviewed 41 patients who had just undergone angioplasties to unclog arteries. Those who scored highest in hostility, described as "Hostile Type A," were 2.5 times more likely to need repeat angioplasty within the year. Hostile Type A behavior has all the same traits as a Type A personality, with the added feature of being angry and hard to get along with. Other studies of people exhibiting the Hostile Type A personality have shown that they have higher levels of adrenaline and stress hormones in their blood, making their vessels more likely to constrict.

ADDICTION

Peter is in his mid-30s and is worried about his alcohol consumption. He denies being an alcoholic and describes himself as a "social drinker" who only drinks beer and wine. Peter has smoked since the age of 12 and has tried to quit numerous times. His average consumption of coffee is about ten cups a day. Peter is hoping his doctor can give him some sort of guidance.

Addiction is an enslaving, destructive dependency; it is like being under the spell of an activity or substance that is psychologically or physically habit-forming, such as narcotics, alcohol, or tobacco, to such an extent that attempting to break free of the dependency causes a severe physical or mental inability to function. Individuals can be physically predisposed to an addiction, and because of the usual medical complications that accompany the problem, addictions are often viewed as diseases. Not all drug addictions involve illegal products. We know, for example, that the two most addictive products, tobacco and alcohol, are limited only by the age of the consumer, are sold in many food stores, and are as easy to purchase as a bottle of milk.

Consider, too, prescription drugs and even certain over-the-counter products. Mood-altering medications account for some of our most obvious addictions. They create physical, emotional, and social dependence on artificially induced feelings. Some stimulants produce an exhilaration that creates an illusion of well-being, power, adequacy, and control. Depressants, such as tranquilizers, can temporarily relieve our anxieties, fears, and inhibitions.

Addictions and Serotonin

Serotonin levels are increased during the intake of addictive substances, such as alcohol, tobacco, certain narcotics, and caffeine. When individuals attempt to kick these habits, they often develop a chemical withdrawal syndrome when Serotonin levels plummet. These findings have been demonstrated and observed in both experimental animals and in people. During withdrawal, patients get the "munchies" and it is known that overeating is, in part, related to chemical dependency withdrawal, a response to low Serotonin levels. These same low Serotonin levels may also be partly related to the severe depression and sleep deprivation that occur during withdrawal. Low Serotonin levels then make the withdrawing addict more prone to use other addictive substances as the body tries to compensate for its Serotonin loss.

Serotonin levels are increased during the intake of addictive substances, such as alcohol, tobacco, certain narcotics, and caffeine. When individuals attempt to kick these habits, they often develop a chemical withdrawal syndrome when serotonin levels plummet.

For example, one group of rats was fed a typical teenage 'junk food" diet. Theses rats continuously increased their alcohol consumption during the study. The second group received a well-balanced control diet. These rats maintained a low level of alcohol intake. When their diets were supplemented with either caffeine or coffee, both groups significantly increased their alcohol intake. Results suggest that "metabolic controls to drinking exist that are sensitive to dietary factors."

Instead of Peter's usual fast-food diet, his doctor put him on a whole foods eating plan, low in sugar and processed foods, and rich in fruits, vegetables, and whole grains. He also told Peter that he would have to greatly reduce his coffee intake down to one or two cups a day and add a high potency, comprehensive multivitamin and mineral supplement. Since Peter felt the urge to drink more in the evening, his doctor had him slowly work up to 100 mg of 5-HTP before dinner. Peter has not only lost weight but his urge to drink has been greatly decreased. He has also stopped smoking after completing a nicotine addiction program.

In a similar study, Purdue University researchers found that consuming alcohol increased the physical craving to smoke. "We've long known that alcohol drinkers smoke more, but this is the first study that actually shows that alcohol physically drives up one's craving to smoke," says Stephen Tiffany, professor of psychological sciences. Study subjects all were told they were drinking alcohol, but only half were actually given real drinks. Those who consumed alcohol had an average 35% increase in their craving to smoke, compared to those participants who received nonalcoholic drinks. Smoking cravings were measured both by questionnaires filled out by the participants and by physical data. "So the impact of the alcohol was pharmacological in nature, not due to their expectations," Tiffany says. He says smokers are highly practiced at their habit, and lighting up when they drink becomes automatic. "Now we know that once they start drinking, their craving to smoke also increases. We did not find evidence that alcohol made people hypersensitive to smoking cues. Instead, consuming alcohol had an additive effect, acting to increase the intensity of the urge that was already present," Tiffany says.

Pain sensitivity also increases when brain Serotonin levels are low. This has been presented by researchers as one contributing factor in premenstrual syndrome (PMS) and in cancer-related pain. Agitation, pain, irritability, and depression, all characteristic aspects of PMS, are reduced markedly by alcohol ingestion, which temporarily increases Serotonin levels in the brain.

Although no one has yet made an argument that Serotonin or 5-HTP can cure addictions, there appears to be mounting evidence that it can reduce the symptoms of withdrawal considerably, giving other treatment modalities a better chance of succeeding.

Drug Addiction and Serotonin

Dr. Rene Hen of Columbia University found "the first

definitive evidence for the involvement of a specific Serotonin receptor in processes that may underlie cocaine addiction." Previous studies had suggested that Serotonin activity affects an individual's response to drugs of abuse, although the exact nature of this role has yet to be clarified. To study the effect of this neurotransmitter, researchers bred a strain of mice lacking one of the brain's receptors for Serotonin, called the 5-receptor. These genetically altered mice are referred to as knockout (KO) mice. These 5-HT receptor-deficient mice learned to self-administer cocaine more quickly than normal mice and exhibited different behavioral responses to the drug. The behavior of the knockout mice was "like that shown by (normal) mice sensitized by repeated exposure to cocaine," the authors summarize. In knockout mice, they also found several biochemical alterations that have been associated with cocaine sensitization in previous research.

An additional 14 million Americans ages 18 and older suffer from alcoholism, and the starting age for alcohol ingestion and addiction is dropping precipitously almost daily. Cases of substance abuse are often complicated by depression, schizophrenia, sexual abuse, personality disorders, or other mental illnesses. And these addiction statistics say nothing of the millions of people legally addicted to tobacco products, which are responsible for more American deaths each year.

Tobacco kills more Americans each year than all of the combined drug, alcohol, accidental, murder, suicide, and war deaths the world over. Add to these numbers the millions of people some authorities consider to be addicted to overeating, gambling, work, and sex and we discover that a frightening percentage of our population is under the control of some outside, demon-like influence. The toll in lost lives and money is astronomical, and the destruction of families and disruption of society is incalculable.

Alcohol and Serotonin

Some aspects of drinking alcohol may be governed by Serotonin neurotransmitter systems. Lab animals that prefer ethanol show a decrease in Serotonin receptor densities and Serotonin function. Selective Serotonin reuptake inhibitors decrease alcohol consumption in animal models. In one study, mice were given one of three SSRis: fluoxetine, sertraline, or paroxetine. The mice were taught how to press a lever and were then given access to a lever that dispensed a drink of ethanol. Initially, all three drugs decreased the amount of times the mice pressed the alcohol lever. Although this effect only lasted a few days and subsequent higher doses of the SSIU were ineffective, the SSRis were again effective after a several week wash-out period. It may be that 5-HTP is only beneficial hardcore drug users in America today: 2.1 million cocaine users and about 600,000 heroin users, as reported in 1994 by the U.S. Office of Drug Control Strategy. An additional 14 million Americans ages 18 and older suffer from alcoholism, and the starting age for alcohol ingestion and addiction is dropping precipitously almost daily. Cases of substance abuse are often complicated by depression, schizophrenia, sexual abuse, personality disorders, or other mental illnesses.

Since Peter felt the urge to drink more in the evening, his doctor had him slowly work up to 100 mg of 5-HTP before dinner. Peter has not only lost weight but his urge to drink has been greatly decreased. He has also stopped smoking after completing a nicotine addiction program.

And these addiction statistics say nothing of the millions of people legally addicted to tobacco products, which are responsible for more American deaths each year than all of the combined drug, alcohol, accidental, murder, suicide, and war deaths the world over. Add to these numbers the millions of people some authorities consider to be addicted to overeating, gambling, work, and sex and we discover that a frightening percentage of our population is under the control of some outside, demon-like influence. The toll in lost lives and money is astronomical, and the destruction of families and disruption of society is incalculable. Nearly 20,000 people died in alcohol related traffic accidents last year, about one every half hour. Alcohol-related deaths account for over 40% of all traffic fatalities. More than 1 million of our population were injured in alcohol-related traffic accidents; that's one person every 30 seconds, with 30,000 of those suffering permanent disabilities.

Further statistics indicate that about 10% of all workers abuse drugs and/or alcohol on the job, and these include physicians, lawyers, pilots, police, and people in other hazardous professions in whose hands we often place our lives and safety. Each year employers pay about $10,000 per each abuser in identifiable costs of doing business; these include expenses for lost production, injuries, damaged equipment, insurance, and other disruptions to efficiency. Each smoker in a company costs an employer about $4,000 a year in lost production, illnesses, dam aged equipment, and health and fire insurance. It is estimated that about 65% of all on the job accidents are caused by sub stance abusers. Three times the number of sickness benefits are used by abusers, especially smokers. Abusers file six times more worker's comp claims than do non-addicted workers, and work absences are over 15 times greater among abusers.

In all addictions, whether to alcohol, drugs, sex, work, gambling, or overeating, addicted people lose control of their lives and feel helpless to stop the behavior that they know full well is destroying them. And because each addicted person affects the lives of others, especially spouses and children, there is a "ripple effect," making addiction one of society's most important challenges. Furthermore, addiction all too often leads to other serious social and personal problems, such as crime, divorce, homelessness, disease, domestic violence, other mental illnesses, accidental death, suicide, and murder.

How to Break the Addiction Cycle

It usually takes intervention by family, employers, friends, physicians, or often the courts to get the addict's attention. Court-ordered treatment, financial ruin, loss of employment, loss of health, or loss of relationships are all too often precursors to getting help. Some outside event or intervention must cause the addict to be willing to reach out for whatever psychological, spiritual, or medical help is needed for him to break the grip of the enslaving, destructive dependency.

MEMORY LOSS

Clarence has just entered his seventh decade, and although he is now 70, he has always prided himself on his youthful appearance and outlook. But in the past few years, Clarence's memory has gotten worse. This has frightened him so much that he will not talk about it to his family. He fears that he is developing Alzheimer's disease just like his wife, who must now live in a nursing home. Without telling his children, and fearing the worst, Clarence makes an appointment with his doctor.

We all notice, from time to time, that we tend to forget, misplace, confuse, or misstate things. We call our kids by their siblings' names, and once in a not-so-seldom while, we forget a name, especially when we are trying to introduce its owner. This usually happens at the most embarrassing times. And our forgetfulness seems to occur more frequently as we age. From the ages of 40 or 45 onward, our first reaction to these lapses of memory is that mentally we are on a downhill slide and Alzheimer's is awaiting us. We've all heard that "you can't teach an old dog new tricks!" Just what happens to the aging mind? Why do we forget? Why can't we keep on learning? When does memory quit and senility begin?

Well, get ready for a little surprise! The aging mind can actually learn easier than the young mind, it reasons far better than a young person's, and it can remember just as well. Furthermore, Alzheimer's affects a very small percentage of our population. Over 100 problems can mimic Alzheimer's and can cause mis-diagnosis, and most of these problems are curable. Fortunately, memory loss and age are not necessarily related and the aging mind can be as sharp as ever. As we age, our memory does not have to suffer. You don't believe it? Let's look at a couple of facts: The average age of all Supreme Court justices is 72 and the average age of Fortune 500 CEOs is 62.

Nutrition and Cognitive Performance

What we eat and drink has an effect on how we think and act. Even short-term fasting has a small but significant effect on intellectual performance. Nutrition becomes even more important as we get older because of age-related changes in the body. As we grow older, our gastrointestinal systems are less able to digest food and absorb nutrients and a lifetime of bad habits eventually take their toll. For example, research shows that a lifetime of having high blood pressure causes shrinkage of the brain.

Well, get ready for a little surprise! The aging mind can actually learn easier than the young mind, it reasons far better than a young person's, and it well. Furthermore, Alzheimer's affects a small a very small percentage of our population.

The Serotonin system also declines with age, according to research performed at the University of Pittsburgh Medical Center. Chief researcher Dr. Carolyn Meltzer found a 55% decrease in Serotonin receptors. This study confirmed the earlier smaller study done by Belgian researchers using a narrower age range of subjects and postmortem reports.

The Role of Serotonin in the Brain

English researchers from the University of Oxford examined the effects of tryptophan on human cognitive performance. Twelve participants were given a low-tryptophan drink to decrease levels of plasma and total free tryptophan. Participants were then given computerized tests measuring memory, learning, and executive function. Tests revealed impairments in cognitive performance. In one test the low-tryptophan drink lengthened thinking time only in subjects already familiar with the task, suggesting a problem in retrieving learned information.

5-HTP and the Brain

Supplemental 5-hydroxy-tryptophan has been found to increase spatial memory in rats. When researchers at Haifa University in Israel gave old rats the 5-HTP, the learnig problems associated with age-dependent spatial learning deficits were decreased. The Israeli researchers hypothesized that it is the Serotonin system that is damaged in aged rats. They noted that "5-HTP appears to be a principal key in helping to maintain and restore spatial memory function." Young rats also benefited from small doses of 5-HTP, although not as much as the aged rats.

Let's return to Clarence and his memory problem.

Clarence's doctor ran some tests on him and concluded that he was healthy. Since Clarence had smoked for many years and also had drug controlled hypertension, the doctor explained that these risk factors were still going to haunt his old age. The first thing Clarence's doctor explained was that his diet was far from optimal. His doctor recommended a high potency vitamin and mineral supplement to supply the B-vitamins needed to transform the amino acids into neurotransmitters. He also wanted him to take 5-HTP to provide the body with the raw material to make Serotonin. Clarence followed his new diet and faithfully took his 100 mg of 5-HTP before bed every night. At his next physical a year later, Clarence reported that his memory was much better. "Maybe it's because I'm sleeping better," he said, "but I never forget to take my 5-HTP."

How Human Memory Works

Human memory is associative, meaning that our brain links different pieces of information together, which form a complex knowledge structure. Our human brain works like a huge information network where the associations can change very quickly. We 've all been in a situation where it was very important for us to remember something, but the harder we tried to remember, the harder it became to access the memory, the stored information. Perhaps the reason for this may have been the loss of a link to a specific piece of information, or maybe our mental lapse was caused by the stress of the moment. The problem wasn't that we forgot or lost the information. It was still stored in our filing cabinet, or brain, or else we never could have recovered it. The problem was that we misfiled it. We hadn't forgotten the data, we'd merely misplaced it.

The human memory also has different stages: ultra-short term memory, short-term memory, and long-term memory. The first time you hear a name, you may hardly pay attention to it, and if you are asked to repeat it even a few seconds later, it just won't be there. Because you paid it so little attention initially, it was stored in the ultra-short-term memory. But once you were caught forgetting it and perhaps were a little embarrassed as a result, the second time you hear the name it will probably stick ... for at least a little while. Now it's filed in the short-term section of your memory file. If you meet that person again and again, the name gets recalled over and over a few times, and it will go into the long-term memory file. Each time it gets "up graded," it becomes easier and easier to recall. "Practice makes perfect!" The trouble with us older folks is that we don't like to practice. We've become unfocused, and we don't pay as much attention to detail as we did when we were young and everything was new and exciting.

Depression closely mimics Alzheimer's disease and is often mis-diagnosed. The benefits of using 5-HTP to alleviate depression have been well-documented.

Forgetting has its useful function, too. Since there is no need for everything to be stored in our brains, the different stages of human memory help to filter out what isn't too important. Since important things get used or thought about more, those are the things that get upgraded to longer-term memories. This helps to protect us from the flood of information coming our way every day, every hour, every minute!

Short-term memory is mediated by a chemical synapse via a neurotransmitter called acetylcholine. It is short-lived if it is not reinforced rather soon after the initial triggering event has occurred. Long-term memory develops when repetition or emotional importance bring about a structural change that actually "cements" the neural pathway chemically, solders the chemical "flux" through repetition. Protein is actually laid down to create a permanent "bridge" to the memory. Thus, repeating a thought or a recall changes the chemical synapse to an actual structural "encoding bridge." If you frequently repeat what you want to remember, you will remember! Rhymes and mnemonics help to encode memories by association. Writing also helps you to encode. Often, just the act of writing a list helps you to remember the items on it. Have you ever made a grocery list that you accidentally left at home, had no choice but to go shopping anyway, and when you got home to check the list you discovered that you had managed to buy nearly everything you'd originally listed ... and usually more?

Retrieval of information becomes easier if attention was paid and either repetition or emotional impact enhanced the initial experience, enabling the brain to encode the new information properly. Then it becomes a matter of finding it in its proper file. Did you ever panic, thinking you had lost a day's work in your computer and then happily find that it had just been misfiled and was actually stored in the wrong place but was still totally intact? That's what usually happens in your brain when you think you've forgotten something. It's almost always there if you can just find it. Try to retrace your steps. Think about what you were doing when you had the experience you were trying to remember. If you were carrying in groceries the last time you had your keys, look in the kitchen to find them! Learn to relax when seeking a memory; adrenaline tend to wipes out memory. Reconstruct situations or scenes. Tie it to other memories and picture what you are trying to remember.

Misdiagnosing Alzheimer's

Things do indeed go wrong at times, but not as often as we are led to believe. Less than 15% of elderly people have actual memory loss and only half of those cases are due to real organic disease. There are over a hundred disorders that can mimic Alzheimer's, causing considerable misdiagnosis of that disease. Here are a few of the most common- and curable- Alzheimer's like conditions.

1. Loneliness and boredom have become too big a part of too many elderly people's days. From loneliness and boredom comes a loss of interest in the environment, in the self, and in life itself. People who have no interest in the world around them often take on the demeanor of a person with organic mental deterioration. Furthermore, these people often eat poorly, having little interest in food. Their diet is frequently low in protein and this can lead to reduced tryptophan and thus low levels of Serotonin, which can impair memory and cause

depression. This physical degeneration worsens their mental state even further. Supplements of 5- HTP may be helpful in these cases.

2. Depression and old age often go hand in hand, as a result of people's loneliness, boredom, or diet. Depression closely mimics Alzheimer's disease and is often misdiagnosed. The benefits of using 5-HTP to alleviate depression have been well-documented.

3. Dehydration of 10% or more frequently produces Alzheimer's-like symptoms. Most elderly people's bodies are up to 15% dehydrated from time to time. Elderly people liv ing alone often neglect the oral intake of fluids, and the sit uation is not much better in nursing homes and assisted living facilities. Nutritional guidance and 5-HTP supplementation would benefit most of these folks.

4. Prescription and over-the-counter drugs can dull an elderly person's personality and will to be active, and can cause lethargic mental processes, to again mimic Alzheimer's disease. The average healthy elderly adult takes five pills per day. The average ill elderly adult takes 11 pills per day. Too many nursing homes feel that a tranquilized patient is a good patient and thus distribute drugs to dull their senses and their sense. All medications should be reviewed with a physician periodically and those that are not absolutely necessary should be stopped.

5. Nutritional deficiency among adults is not only a result of other problems such as depression, but it is often a primary problem and can, on its own, cause Alzheimer's-like 1 symptoms. Frequently, it is "too much trouble" to fix a

nourishing meal for oneself, so meals are skipped or replaced by high-carbohydrate snacks. This can cause protein deficiency and low serotonin levels, leading to further depression. Taking 5-HTP and vitamin supplements would be beneficial to these people.

The good news is that these problems and the hundred others that can mimic Alzheimer's disease are all reversible if the causative deficiency is replaced. The diagnosis of Alzheimer's should not be made until all other possible causes for the symptoms have been ruled out.

Whoever came up with the saying "You can't teach old dogs new tricks!" as a metaphor for the learning abilities of the elderly was way off. The fact of the matter is that if motivated the elderly can actually learn faster and better than the young.

Alzheimer's Disease

The Alzheimer's diagnosis may not always be correct, but too often it is. It is a devastating disease, an irreversible cause of dementia in older people. Dementia is a medical condition that disrupts the way the brain works. Alzheimer's disease affects the parts of the brain that control thought, memory, and language. To date, the cause of the disease is still unknown and there is no cure. An estimated 4 million people in the United States suffer from Alzheimer's disease. Its onset usually begins after age 65, and the risk of contracting it goes up with age. While younger people may also get Alzheimer's, this is much less common. About 3% of men and women ages 65 to 74 have Alzheimer's, but the disease is not a normal part of the aging process.

Scientists have found significant changes in the brains of people with Alzheimer's. There is a loss of nerve cells in areas of the brain that are vital to memory and other mental abilities.

There are lower levels of chemicals in the brain that carry complex messages between billions of nerve cells. The disease may disrupt normal thinking and memory by not letting these messages between nerve cells get through.

Symptoms

Alzheimer's disease begins slowly, with the only symptom being mild forgetfulness. People may have trouble remembering recent events, activities, or the names of familiar people or things. Simple math problems may become hard to solve. Such difficulties may be a bother, but usually they are not serious enough to cause alarm.

As the disease goes on, symptoms are more easily noticed and become acute enough to cause the individuals or their family members to seek medical help. People with the disease may forget how to do simple tasks, such as brushing their teeth, combing their hair, or expressing themselves. They can no longer think clearly and begin to have problems speaking, understanding, reading, or writing. Later on, they may become anxious or aggressive or wander away from home. Eventually, they may require total care. Doctors at specialized centers can correctly diagnose probable Alzheimer's disease 80% to 90% of the time.

Treatment

Alzheimer's disease is a slow, progressive disease, starting with mild memory problems and ending with severe mental damage. How long a course the disease takes and how fast changes occur vary from person to person and may run from five to twenty or more years. To date, there is no treatment that can stop the disease. However, for some people in the early and middle stages of the disease, the drugs Tacrine, or THAT, or

Cognex may alleviate some symptoms. Also, certain medicines may help to control behavioral symptoms of Alzheimer's disease, such as sleeplessness, agitation, wandering, anxiety, and depression. Treating these symptoms often makes patients more comfortable and makes their care easier for care-givers. Supplemental 5-HTP has been used in Europe for some of these secondary symptoms with a degree of success.

Most often, spouses or other family members provide the day-to-day care for people with Alzheimer's. This can be hard for care-givers and can affect their physical and mental health, family life, jobs, and finances. Supplements of 5-HTP may be a good stabilizing agent for these care-givers, balancing their moods without slowing their faculties, easing the depression that attends their efforts, and helping them get much-needed rest at night. Perhaps the most immediate effect of 5-HTP is its ability to induce sleep when taken on an empty stomach about one hour before going to bed. A 100- mg dose is adequate to induce sleep in a large adult male. Both 5-HTP and Serotonin (5-HT) are precursors to another neurotransmitter-melatonin that also induces sleep. Using it to help agitated Alzheimer's patients fall asleep is also practical.

Learning New Tricks

Whoever came up with the saying "You can't teach old dogs new tricks!" as a metaphor for the learning abilities of the elderly was way off. The fact of the matter is that, if motivated, the elderly can actually learn faster and better than the young. To maintain my skills and credentials to continue working as an emergency room physician, I, at 75, had to continue to take courses to update my knowledge and recertify my eligibility and maintain my medical license yearly. The physicians who take these recertification and updating programs with me range in age from their mid-20s to their late 60s and 70s. Compared to the young doctors, we "old-timers" pick up the new material as easily, if not more so, than the "upstarts." Have you taken a hard look at college campuses lately? You'll see lots of us old folks ... grandmothers, grandfathers, even great-grandparents ... sitting in classes. Seldom are we at the bottom of the class, and we come by the knowledge of the material rather easily. It's because we have a wealth of foundation knowledge gained by years of experience, reading, study, and work. Much learning is a reorganization of old material; thus, we who have experience have an advantage.

It's the lack of motivation that keeps us from learning new material. Old dogs would rather sleep by the fire and watch the pups learn to roll over. But great rewards are to be had by learning new tricks. We can develop satisfying hobbes or even start new and exciting careers by learning new tricks. Master all ... if we're going to outlive all of our ancestors' lifespans, we might as well stay active enough to enjoy those added years.

Apathy to Atrophy . . .
Stimulation to Sharpness!

As with the muscles of the body, disuse of the mind will cause atrophy . . . but stimulation of the brain can stop the mental atrophy and then reverse the process to growth and more effective mental functioning. How often do active, bright people reach the age of 65 and then retire from a job that had kept them sharp and on their toes, only to deteriorate over the next year or so into a nursing home or the grave? It happens all the time. You have to exercise the body to keep it in good physical shape and you have to exercise the mind to keep it mentally sharp. You must realign your priorities for your next lifestyle change not retirement, but new ventures to broaden your horizons and interests, pursuits and experiences. Seek out activities, adult education, travel, reading, writing, music, hobbies, nature, and all of the things you wanted to do but never had the time for. Use it and you won't lose it! Get creative! Get involved with organizations that need your help or seek help from groups that are out there to help you become creative and inventive and exercise the mind. These organizations include Elderhostel, AARP, the YMCA, community programs, church programs, art programs, writing clubs, and travel clubs.

Some Activities to Keep You Healthy in Mind and Body

An avocation that requires skill development and concentration on detail is the best thing to keep your mind active and developing. In seeking avocations that are best suited to you, try several activities and continue with those that are enjoyable and challenging. Perhaps a good place to start is to think about some of the things you wanted to do when you were younger but didn't have the time or finances to pursue.

As an added benefit, when you achieve proficiency in your avocation, it will go a long way toward boosting your selfesteem. If you can't think of a niche for yourself, the following suggestions may help:

Exercise Team sports, tennis, golf, hiking, bodybuilding, swimming, and gardening are all activities that fit into this category.

Travel A vacation is a great revitalizer. The main problem is that we can't usually take enough of them. As wonderful as it is to get away for two weeks or longer, frequent long weekends are probably better for us. If you only get two weeks' vacation, ten working days, you may do better by using them around holiday weekends and getting several four or five day trips a year.

Bowling As a game of skill and a way to get out with people and take your mind off distressing problems, bowling has plenty going for it. You can join a league, adding excite ment and good fellowship ... or you can just challenge yourself with constant improvement.

Music "Music tames the savage beast!" There may be no truer statement. Perhaps that is why many conductors, composers and musicians can remain active into their late 80s and 90s. Here, I'm not suggesting that you be only a spectator. You're never too old to take music lessons. Perhaps you did take lessons but didn't pursue music as far as you'd have liked. There's no better time than the present to remedy that mistake. The study of music is one of the most mind stimulating activities you can find.

Camping This is a fun and challenging way to travel and meet new and interesting people. You can back-pack in, or you can drive to the thousands of campgrounds throughout the world. You can buy or rent a recreational vehicle and have the freedom of a modern-day Gypsy. You might try taking a wilderness course to develop some real survival skills.

Carpentry If you are talented with your hands and have a creative urge, consider carpentry or model-building. What can be more satisfying and distress-reducing than to see your own creations come to life as you build with woods and tools?

Painting Watercolors, oils, acrylics, chalk, crayons, pencils, ink, and charcoal all await you to give them a try. You may never sell a picture, but that isn't the main purpose. There are few activities that can be more absorbing than to dabble in paint, color, form. . . .

Sculpture Who didn't enjoy modeling clay as a child? Why not try the adult version? Sculpture, ceramics, origami, welding, carving, and papier-mache are just a few of the ways for you to create in three dimensions.

Reading No matter what other avocation you may choose, there are times when nothing beats a good book in which to lose yourself. Create time for yourself to get through some of those books you didn't have time for in the past. Reading is always a mind-stimulating activity.

Writing As a writer I can tell you firsthand, there is no more forgiving art form than writing. Anyone can do it! And just about everyone has said at one time or another, "I'd like to write a book about ..." Well, there's no time like the present to get started. Writing especially activates memory and recall.

Gardening Gardening can be a wonderful avocation and any one can get into it. You can get started with just a few pots and plants or even seeds. Gardening can be scaled to your own space and needs. There is no end to how far you can take this hobby. You can specialize in orchids, roses, cacti, succulents, wild flowers, herbs, vegetables, trees, fruits, shrubs, or you can go for it all. Get a little dirt under your nails and give it a fair try.

Volunteer Work There is perhaps no more satisfying avocation than volunteer work. Helping others who are less fortunate than we are has its own rewards. It's a way of paying back for our own good fortune and blessings. Try giving a few hours of yourself a week and see what it does to your distress and anger levels. You are a valuable commodity and resource, and you owe it to yourself and your community, your world, to share yourself with others. Nothing will do more for your self-esteem than to know you've helped others who are much worse off than you are.

Hiking If you are near the woods, mountains, lakes, rivers, countryside, or anywhere else that lends itself to hiking, then, by all means, hike. It's an avocation in which you can participate with your spouse, the whole family, grand children, and friends. Notice the animals and birds, plants and trees. Even insects can be fascinating. Observe nature and try to learn about it. Here's an opportunity to slow down and see things that you've been too busy and too rushed to enjoy in years past.

Teaching In all the years you've lived and experienced, you've learned a lot more than you realize. You have skills and knowledge that others can and want to learn from. Teaching is one of the most satisfying and fun experiences you can imagine. Check around your local schools and universities. Many have adult continuing education programs that offer any number of courses, from ballroom dancing to word processing, bookkeeping, languages, entrepreneur ship, and writing.

Golf Golf, like bowling, deserves special mention. It is a skilled activity that constantly challenges you and is an excellent hobby. It takes you out of doors, expands your friendships, is something you can do with friends and acquaintances, is mind-absorbing, and does help you to stay physically limber. If you can walk the course, all the better.

FishingFishing is an international pastime. You can practice this art anywhere in the world. From trolling to fly-casting to deep sea fishing and spear fishing, it's always a challenge. You can get a workout fishing or you can snooze on the bank of a stream or lake waiting for a strike, but whichever you do, it is a good distress-reducing activity. Fishing is a great family avocation, or you can sneak off by yourself if solitude is what you need.

Photography Photography is an activity that works in combination with almost any other hobby you might choose. With today's amazing and amazingly inexpensive automatic cameras, almost anyone can be an expert photographer. And with the easy-to-use video cameras, you can even be your own movie producer.

LearningToday there are so many adult education courses offered by public schools, colleges, churches, synagogues, organizations, museums, galleries, and private institutions that you can study almost anything you want. Learning, in and of itself, is a wonderful hobby, but, more importantly, it can intraduce you to many other exciting activities and interests to pursue in the future. You can even take courses over the Internet, but I suggest you get out into classes where you can make new acquaintances.

DancingBallroom dancing is making a real comeback these days, with competitions and clubs popping up everywhere. Or maybe you just want to be able to "cut a mean rug" once in a while at parties or on nights out. Dancing is a very healthy avocation, giving you a good workout while taking your mind off disturbing factors in your life.

Biking If you have good bike paths available to you, give it a try. You should be able to rent a bike to give it a fair trial before investing in your own.

This listing is just a scratch on the surface of all the leisure time activities you can get involved in. The most important thing is that you get involved. Don't limit yourself to just one avocation. The more activities you engage in, the broader your interests will be and the better and more relaxed you'll feel for it. *Meet new friends, challenge your mind, and enjoy life!*

Vivid Memories

There are some memories that just won't go away, even though the experience that they recall happened to us only once and perhaps fleetingly. We experience a moment's terror and its memory stays to haunt us, or we have a joyous moment and it continues to delight us each time we recall it. Both experiences may have only taken an instant of time, yet they are as vivid as the moment we experienced them-sometimes we feel they are even *more* vivid. It seems that emotional experiences help to "cement" their memories into the brain. Memories are saved on different levels, with some staying in the brain for only a few seconds, with others being retrievable after a degree of effort, while others become permanent, easily recalled, even with no active effort on our part; they are triggered automatically by a sound, a fragrance, or a similar situation.

Also, certain medicines may help to control behavioral symptoms of A Alzheimer's disease, such as sleepless ness, agitation, wandering, anxiety, and depression. Treating these symptoms often makes patients more comfortable and makes their care easier for care-givers. Supplemental 5-HTP has been used in Europe for some of these secondary symptoms with a degree of success.

Important aspects of creating a good memory are: giving proper attention to the event or material to be remembered, encoding the memory for storage, and making the material re trievable when we try to recall it. Again, practice makes perfect. The more we practice a thing, repeat it, think about it, write it, the more attention we give it. And each time we repeat it, the neural pathway carrying the memory gets strengthened and more firmly encoded or changed from a visual or aural or otherwise sensed experience into electronic codes to be stored, in a manner that is not unlike the way your computer stores its information into memory. And the more we practice, the easier it is to recall the material or bring it out of storage.

All of us have a degree of eidetic imagery, which is otherwise known as photographic memory. We all have it if we pay sufficient attention to it. But as it is with our computers, our minds have superior abilities built into them that we don't even know about, much less use. Once we learn about these higher functions and use them a few times, they become second nature to us. Yet instead of applying our attention to the things we may want to remember, with age we tend to day dream more and pay attention less.

HEADACHES

Jennifer has about three sick headaches a month, usually around the time of her period. The pain starts in the back of her neck and then moves to her eye. "It feels like I have a knife in my eye." Once the headache starts, she finds that she cannot tolerate light and even normal sounds hurt her ears and make the throbbing in her head worse. Jennifer deals with the pain by lying down in her bedroom away from light and sound. When she finally sees her doctor, she is surprised that the doctor diagnoses migraine headachs.

Migraine headache is a neurological disorder that is characterized by recurrent attacks, with pain most often occurring on one side of the head, usually accompanied by combinations of symptoms such as nausea, vomiting, sensitivity to light (or photophobia), and sound sensitivity. Migraine headaches can occur at any time of the day or night, but they occur most frequently upon arising in the morning. Routine activity, or even the slightest head movement, typically makes the pain worse. Attacks can last from several hours to several days and are usually disabling. Pain may migrate from one part of the head to another during each episode and may also radiate down the neck into the shoulder; a majority of patients experience scalp tenderness during or after an attack.

Migraine headaches usually occur among family members and they frequently appear to be hereditary, so if you have migraine, chances are another member of your family does as well. Migraine affects over 26 million Americans and can strike at any age; however, it occurs most commonly in young adult women. Following an attack, many individuals feel tired, washed out, irritable, and listless, or they have impaired concentration or an inability to focus. Although migraine is not considered a curable disease, it is usually manageable with proper medical care. Fortunately, a variety of therapies and medications can be helpful. Some reduce or relieve the symptoms, while others reduce the frequency and duration of the headache attacks.

Physiology of Migraine Headaches

In Hippocrates' day, the culprit that supposedly caused migraine headaches was considered to be an excess of yellow or black bile. Today, the evidence implicates Serotonin, changes in the size of blood vessels, and the activity of nerve fibers that relay sensory signals. Serotonin, as we've seen, has a broad spectrum of actions. It influences the tissues in which it is synthesized and stimulates and interacts with various types of receptors on individual target tissues.

But Serotonin is just half of the picture. The various receptors and their responses are equally important. These receptors are specific proteins on the surface of the tissue to which the Serotonin binds, thus triggering certain biological responses in the body. Several types of Serotonin receptors have been identified throughout the body. The body's reaction to serotonin is directly related to the nature of the specific type of Serotonin receptor that is activated. In other words, different receptors react differently to Serotonin mediation and stimulation.

Recent Serotonin research has led to the development of medications that are selectively designed to activate Serotonin's activity (known as Serotonin agonists) or to block Serotonin's action (known as Serotonin antagonists). The Serotonin receptors are numbered to label them according to their reaction to Serotonin stimulation. The Serotonin-!receptor, a specific receptor that is thought to be involved in migraine headaches, is found primarily in the cranial blood vessels and nerves. During a migraine attack, it is thought that the Serotonin level decreases, allowing blood vessels to dilate. This sequence causes surrounding tissues to swell, including the nerve endings that transmit impulses to the brain, which results in the throbbing pain of migraine. As migraine symptoms worsen, Serotonin levels decrease. Intracranial blood vessels dilate, resulting in a decrease in blood flow. Left alone, symptoms improve and the attack stops by the return of Serotonin synthesis.

Migraine Treatment

Stimulation of Serotonin-I type receptors by medications hastens recovery. In the early 1990s the medication Imitrex, or sumatriptan, became available. It is the only selective agonist specifically targeted for the Serotonin-1 receptor. As a Serotonin-1 agonist, it mimics the action of Serotonin at the Serotonin-1 receptor site, constricting the dilated blood vessels and relaxing the pain and associated symptoms. Imitrex is indicated for the treatment of acute migraine attacks, but it should only be used when a clear diagnosis of migraine has been established. In some people, SSRis have also been effective in preventing migraines.

5-HTP and Migraine

In migraine, there is a need to increase Serotonin or stimulate Serotonin type-1 receptors and to block or lower dopamine. Supplements of 5-HTP may help by making the Serotonin precursor available. A few studies have found that 5-HTP may also be able to prevent migraines.

Spanish researchers gave either 5-HTP or methysergide, a long-time migraine treatment, to 124 migraine suffers. Sig nificant improvement was noted in 71% of the 5-HTP-treated participants and 75% of the methysergide-treated participants. In those treated with 5-HTP, the improvement took form as reduced intensity and duration, while frequency remained unchanged. Side effects in the 5-HTP group were also lower than side effects in the methysergide group. The authors suggested that 5-HTP could be a treatment of choice in migraine prophylaxis.

A group of Italian researchers con firmed the prophylactic effect of 5- HTP in 40 patients with migraine in a double-blind study. The patients were divided into two groups. One group received 400 mg of 5-HTP a day and the other received a placebo. At the end of two months, the group that received the 5-HTP had more than a 90% reduction in headache severity, frequency, and duration. The placebo group had only a 16% reduction.

Causes of Migraine

The exact cause of migraine headaches is uncertain. One theory is that migraine develops because the nervous system is vulnerable to sudden changes either within the body or in the environment; according to this reasoning, migraine sufferers have inherited a more sensitive nervous system response to such changes than people who are not prone to getting migraine headaches. During a migraine attack, changes in brain activity produce an inflammation of the blood vessels and nerves in and around the brain. Migraine medication may produce relief by quieting sensitive nerve pathways and reducing their inflammatory reactions.

Migraine Management

it is important that therapy be individualized. There are many migraine drugs available today. Some migraine medications are also used to treat other medical conditions, such as the beta-blockers that are prescribed for hypertension and tricyclic antidepressants, often administered for depression; but the benefits of these therapies in migraine are not necessarily related to the treatment of the other conditions.

Some treatments are intended to stop an attack when it occurs and to treat its symptoms, while others, usually prescribed for individuals who experience frequent attacks, are prophylactic or preventive treatments, to be taken regularly so that migraines will occur less often and last for a shorter periods of time.

Targeting Migraine Triggers

If the pattern of migraine attacks suggests a sensitivity to stimuli or to triggers that can be easily avoided, modification of one's lifestyle may be the best treatment. Steps that can be taken to increase resistance to migraine headaches include regular sleep patterns, a healthful diet and regularly scheduled mealtimes, regular exercise, smoking cessation, relaxation, and meditation. Supplemental 5-HTP can be beneficial in helping to establish good sleep habits, since it is also a precursor to melatonin and is thought to have even stronger sleep inducing characteristics than tryptophan has. If a change in eating habits also requires a reduction in food intake, 5-HTP supplements can help to reduce hunger. In the case of giving up smoking, 5-HTP may help reduce the withdrawal symptoms of anxiety, depression, and irritability.

In migraine, there is a need to increase serotonin or stimulate Serotonin type-1 receptors and to block or lower dopamine. Supplements of 5-HTP may help by making the Serotonin precursor available. A few studies have found that 5-HTP may also be able to prevent migraines.

A variety of relaxation techniques can help manage the body's response to life's daily pressures. Learning to pace your activities is of great importance. If you set aside time each day to sit quietly with your eyes closed, let your muscles relax, and give your mind a break, it can defuse tension and disarm stress triggers. Regular physical activity also helps to reduce stress and keeps you on an even keel.

Environmental factors to avoid include glaring sunlight and fluorescent lights, long hours in front of computer screens, exposure to strong odors and other vivid stimuli, and high altitudes.

Triggers of Migraine

Certain factors can provoke or trigger migraine. Not all migraine headaches have the same triggering factors, nor do all these factors always provoke an attack.

Diet

There are a number of dietary triggers that reportedly provoke migraine, and these include: alcohol; wine (especially red wine); foods containing monosodium glutamate, or MSG; foods that contain tyramine, such as aged cheeses; and. preserved meats with nitrates and nitrites. Keeping a food diary is an important tool to help identify migraine triggers.

Sleep

Too much or too little sleep can trigger migraine attacks.

Hormones

Many women who suffer from migraine have attacks that are linked to their menstrual cycles; these headaches are probably caused hormone levels. Menstrual migranes can be more debilitating and difficult to treat, and they can last longer. Also women during early pregnancy may have increased migraines, but then they usually improve in later pregnancy. The attack typically decline with use of oral contraceptives. In some cases estrogen replacement therapy can worsen migraines.

Stress Headaches

Emotional stress or life's daily pressures can trigger a migraine attack in many individuals.

Environmental Factors

Environmental triggers of migraine headaches include weather or temperature changes, glaring sunlight or the irritation of fluorescent lights, computer screens, strong odors, loud noises, vivid colors or other intense stimulation, and high altitude.

FIBROMYALGIA AND
CHRONIC FATIGUE SYNDROME

Julie has just recently been diagnosed with both fibrornyalgia and chronic fatigue syndrome. She has had symptoms of both since childhood. Julie has trouble falling asleep at night and feels extremely stiff and achy in the morning. "I feel just like a truck ran over me." Her rheumatologist has prescribed Prozac for the pain and Elavil, a tricyclic, for deeper sleep. This treatment, while helping marginally, also leaves her groggy and sleepy in the morning. "I feel like I have a hangover." Julie discontinued the treatment and made an appointment with a naturopathic practitioner for an alternative to drug treatment.

Fibromyalgia syndrome, or FMS, is a rheumatic musculo skeletal disorder, the symptoms of which are widespread muscular and connective tissue pain and generalized fatigue; its cause is still unknown. Fibromyalgia actually means pain of the fibrous tissues of the body: the muscles, ligaments, and tendons. FMS used to be called fibrositis, implying that there was inflammation in the muscles and connective tissues, but research has proven otherwise. The majority of patients with fibromyalgia report that they ache all over their bodies. Their muscles twitch, spasm, and at times burn, and generally feel as if they have been over-stretched and overworked. More women than men are afflicted with fibromyalgia and it shows up in people of all ages. The symptoms are not unlike those of a very bad flu, but complete improvement of the condition never seems to occur. Every muscle of the body seems to cry out in pain.

Perhaps worse than the pain, however, is the feeling of being devoid of energy. FMS resembles a post-viral state. Many experts in the field of fibromyalgia syndrome and chronic fatigue syndrome believe that these two illnesses are different spectrums of the same disease process. For the purposes of this book, we will consider them to be a single entity.

Related Syndromes

Fibromyalgia rarely travels alone. It is usually accompanied by a number of overlapping syndromes and symptoms including: an irritated gut (irritable bowel syndrome, esophageal reflux and spasm, difficulty in swallowing), irritated bladder, dry eyes and mouth, vasoconstriction in the extremities (Raynaud's phenomena), vasoconstriction in the skin (livido reticularis), migraine, photophobia, myofascial pain syndrome, and sleep disorders. And this is the short list! Many of the symptoms appear to be caused by either neurotransmitter imbalance or inappropriate muscle contraction.

More women than men are afflicted with fibromyalgia and it shows up in people of all ages. The symptoms are not unlike those of a very bad flu, but complete improvement of the condition never seems to occur. Every muscle of the body seems to cry out in pain. Perhaps worse than the pain, however, is the feeling of being devoid of energy. FMS resembles a post-viral state.

Who Gets Fibromyalgia?

Contrary to the popular stereotype, fibromyalgia is not "the new yuppie flu." It actually has a very long history ... it has been around long before the yuppies came on the scene. Clinical portraits of diseases similar to CFS have been reported under different medical guises for more than a century. In the 1860s,

Dr. George Beard named the syndrome *neurasthenia*, believing it to be a neurosis that was characterized by weakness and chronic fatigue. Succeeding generations have favored different explanations, such as iron-poor blood, hypoglycemia, environmental allergy, or hypersensitivity to yeast.

In the late 1980s the modern stereotype arose because those who sought help for and stimulated scientific interest in fibromyalgia, or chronic fatigue syndrome, were mostly well educated and affluent women in their mid-30s and 40s. Although it afflicts women more then men, CFS/FMS is now seen in people of all ages, races, professions, and socio economic classes, and in countries around the world.

The Cause of Fibromyalgia or Chronic Fatigue Syndrome

The cause or causes of fibromyalgia and chronic fatigue syndrome remain elusive and baffling. There are, however, suspected triggering events that seem to precipitate the syndrome's onset. Among these triggers are viral or bacterial infections, accidents, or the onset of another unrelated disorder such as rheumatoid arthritis, lupus, or hypothyroidism. Triggering events aren't the cause of FMS, but they seem to awaken an underlying genetic or physiological abnormality that is already present and that predisposes one to the disease.

Theories pertaining to alterations in neurotransmitter regulation, particularly serotonin and norepinephrine, and immune system functions, sleep physiology, hormonal control, and substance P are all under serious investigation in numerous labs all over the world. Substance P is a pain neurotransmitter that has been found to be elevated to three times the normal level in the spinal fluid of fibromyalgia patients.

Tryptophan

Since Serotonin dysfunction seems to be one of the major disturbances in people with fibromyalgia, it only seems natural that tryptophan would be used to treat it. Tryptophan's main effect is to promote the deep sleep that is so absent in this syndrome. However, there is one concern. A few reports suggest that people with fibromyalgia may metabolize tryptophan unevenly. In the normal person, tryptophan can be either metabolized into 5-HTP or kynurenine. In persons suffering from CFS/FMS, not enough tryptophan is made into 5-HTP. There is some concern about "over-feeding" the kynurenine pathway with more tryptophan, thus further elevating its levels.

Serotonin and CFS/FMS

Patients with CFS/FMS have low Serotonin levels in the brain. Systemically, Serotonin is normally stored in the blood platelets. However, a few reports suggest that in this syndrome there is a platelet storage defect. The platelets will not hold onto Serotonin and, consequently, platelet levels in the body are low while Serotonin serum levels are high. The effect of low brain levels of Serotonin are known, pain, migraine, insomnia, depression, and anxiety. The effect of high serum Serotonin levels in the blood is as yet unknown.

Contrary to the popular stereotype, fibromyalgia is not "the new yuppie flu." It actually has a very long history ... it has been around long before the yuppies came on the scene. Clinical portraits of diseases similar to CFS have been reported under different medical guises for more than a century.

Cortisol levels also appear to be elevated in this syndrome, while growth hormone levels are decreased. Cortisol is a hormone secreted as a result of the fight or flight reaction. This puts those with CFS/FMS in a chronic stage of alert. Since high cortisol levels also inhibit the formation of Serotonin from tryptophan, this may in part explain low Serotonin levels.

CFS/FMS is notorious for causing a sleep disorder where stage 3 sleep intrudes into stage 4 sleep. This causes the all too familiar morning sensation of being "run over by a truck." Fibromyalgia researchers call it "non-refreshing sleep." Without sufficient stage 4 sleep, growth hormone cannot be produced. Without growth hormone, the cells of the body cannot be properly maintained. This may account for the exaggerated fatigue experienced after exertion. The muscle cells never get the opportunity to completely heal after normal wear and tear. Serotonin is not the only neurotransmitter imbalance in those with CFS/FMS, but many of the symptoms can be moderated by increasing its levels.

5-HTP

By supplying the body with 5-HTP instead of tryptophan, you are assured that all of the supplement will feed the Serotonin pathway. You no longer have to worry about high cortisol levels inhibiting the formation of 5-HTP from tryptophan.

For a minute, let us return to the case of Julie from the beginning of this chapter. Julie was unable to continue treatment because of the side effects of the drugs.

After Julie was examined by her naturopath, he explained that both the pain and lack of deep sleep were the result of a Serotonin dysfunction. He recommended that Julie start on 5-HTP, to be taken every evening before bed. To start, Julie took a low dose of only 20 mg. This was, he explained, because people with fibromyalgia are very sensitive to drugs.

After three days Julie increased the dose to 50 mg and over the course of two weeks to 150 mg. Almost immediately, Julie noticed an increase in the amount of refreshing sleep she was able to get. But this time she had no side effects, no drugged feeling. In the morning she hurt less and was less stiff. After a month, Julie5- depression lifted and she found herself better able to handle the emotional pressures a pain syndrome presents.

The use of 5-hydroxy-tryptophan for the treatment of fibromyalgia is becoming more and more commonplace. In one open 90-day study, 5-HTP was given to 50 FMS patients. There was a significant improvement in all the studied symptoms throughout the trial, including a number of tender points, anxiety, pain intensity, quality of sleep, and fatigue. Patient and investigator evaluations indicated a "good to fair" improvement in nearly half of the patients during the 90 days. A total of 15 (30% of patients) reported side effects, but only one patient was withdrawn from the treatment for this reason. Researchers concluded that "5-HTP is effective in improving the symptoms of primary fibromyalgia syndrome and that it maintains its efficacy throughout the 90-day period of treatment."

Sometimes 5-HTP is used in combination with another drug. One study randomly administered a combination of monoamine oxidase inhibitors (MAOis) with 5-HTP, 5-HTP alone, MAO is alone, or the tricyclic drug amitriptyline, in order to compare the effectiveness of these treatments. The combination of MAO is with 5-HTP significantly improved fibromyalgia syndrome while the other treatments yielded fewer benefits.

Treatments

Most treatments today are aimed toward improving the quality of sleep and reducing pain. Because the deep level of stage 4 sleep is so crucial for many important body functions, such as tissue repair, antibody production, and perhaps even the regulation and production or secretion of various neurotransmitters, hormones, and immune system chemicals, the sleep disorders that frequently occur in fibromyalgia and chronic fatigue patients are thought to be a major contributing factor to the symptoms of this condition. Examples of drugs to help sleep commonly pre scribed in fibromyalgia include Elavil, Flexeril, Sinequan, Paxil, Serzone, Xanax, and Klonopin. The nonsteroidal anti-inflammatory drugs, or NSAIDs, such as ibuprofen and Naprosyn, seem at times to be beneficial. Many patients use additional other treatment methods such as malic acid, magnesium, guaifenesin, trigger point injections with lidocaine, physical therapy, acupuncture, acupressure, relaxation techniques, osteopathic manipulation, chiropractic care, therapeutic massage, and gentle exercise programs.

Fibromyalgia is a chronic disease, but the symptoms may ease, go into remission, and then recur. The impact that FMS can have on the activities of daily life differs among patients. A follow-up of people who meet the chronic fatigue syndrome criteria indicates that as many as 40% of them may significantly improve, but that few appear to completely recover from this syndrome.

Diagnosis

Diagnosing FMS or CFS is difficult because of symptoms they share with many other diseases. Physicians must first rule out diseases that look similar to FMS, , for example, diseases such as multiple sclerosis and lupus. To make matters more difficult, it may take years for diagnostic symptoms in these diseases to fully develop. In follow-up visits, physicians need to be alert to any new clues or symptoms that might indicate a diagnosis other than CFS. Only after physicians rigorously exclude people suffering from other diseases can a correct diagnosis be made for the remaining large group of people who have symptoms associated with debilitating fatigue. Based on the first three years of an ongoing surveillance study in four U.S. cities, the CDC estimates that the minimum prevalence rate of CFS in the United States is 4 to 10 cases per 100,000 adults 18 years of age or older.

Symptoms of CFS/FMS

Fibromyalgia, or chronic fatigue syndrome, may take several different routes to reach the state of chronic exhaustion that is exhibited. Perhaps, in some people, a persistent viral infection may provoke the symptoms. Virologists continue to explore this possibility. Vulnerability to fibromyalgia syndrome may be associated with a subtle immune system defect. Genetics may hold the key to determining who is predisposed to this debilitating disease. It also appears likely that CFS involves interactions between the immune and central nervous systems. Obviously, these are interactions about which relatively little is yet known. The important thing is that FMS/ CFS, whichever name you want to call it, has the attention of the scientific community. No longer do patients with this disease have to feel "It's all in the mind!" This is a disease with severe consequences and it needs to be taken very seriously.

Pain- Patients with FMS describe the pain as deep muscular aching, burning, stiffening, throbbing, shooting, and stabbing. Usually, the pain and stiffness are worse in the morning and may hurt more in muscle groups that are used- repetitively.

CFS/FMS is notorious for causing a sleep disorder where stage 3 sleep intrudes into stage 4 sleep. This causes the all too familiar morning sensation of being "run over by a truck." Fibromyalgia researchers call it "nonrefreshing sleep." Without sufficient stage 4 sleep, growth hormone cannot be produced. Without growth hormone, the cells of the body cannot be properly maintained. This may account for the exaggerated fatigue experienced after exertion. The muscle cells never get the opportunity to completely heal after normal wear and tear.

Fatigue - The fatigue symptoms may be mild in some patients and, in others, totally incapacitating. It has been described as feeling as if one's arms and legs are tied to concrete blocks. Furthermore, there is a mental component to the fatigue that causes difficulty concentrating.

Sleep Disorder - Most fibromyalgia patients have an associated sleep disorder known as the alpha-EEG anomaly, which is measurable by recording brain waves during sleep. Researchers found that fibromyalgia syndrome patients could fall asleep without much trouble, but their deep level, or stage 4, sleep was constantly interrupted by repeated bursts of awake-like brain activity. Most patients who have been diagnosed with chronic fatigue syndrome have the same alpha-EEG sleep pattern and some fibromyalgia-diagnosed patients have been found to have other sleep disorders, such as sleep myoclonus, or nighttime jerking of the arms and legs; restless leg syndrome; and bruxism.

Irritable Bowel Syndrome - Constipation, diarrhea, frequent abdominal cramping, flatulence, abdominal bloating, and nausea are symptoms frequently found in up to 70% of fibromyalgia patients.

Headache - Frequent migraine or tension-type headaches are seen in about 50% of fibromyalgia patients.

Temporomandibular Joint Dysfunction Syndrome - This syndrome, sometimes referred to as TMJD, causes tremendous facial and head pain in about 25% of FMS patients. However, a 1997 report indicates that as many as 90% of fibromyalgia patients may have jaw and facial tenderness that could pro duce, at least intermittently, symptoms of TMJD. Most of the problems associated with this condition are thought to be related to the muscles and ligaments surrounding the joints and not necessarily to the joint itself; however, the sleep disorder bruxism, or teeth-grinding during sleep, can cause TMJD as well.

Multiple Chemical Sensitivity Syndrome-Sensitivities to vivid sensations such as strong odors, noise, bright lights, and to many medications and various foods is common in roughly half of FMS or CFS patients.

Other Common Symptoms - Symptoms that most patients will have either intermittently or all the time can include painful menstrual periods, or dysmenorrhea; chest pain; morning stiffness; cognitive or memory impairment; numbness and tingling sensations; muscle twitching; irritable bladder; the feeling of swollen extremities; skin sensitivities; dry eyes and mouth; frequent changes in eyeglass prescription; dizziness; and impaired coordination.

Aggravating Factors - Numerous environmental factors can cause exacerbations of FMS symptoms and these include changes in the weather, cold or drafty environments, seasonal changes, hormonal fluctuations of the body, menstrual and menopausal hormonal changes, distress, depression, anxiety, the onset of other illnesses, and over-exertion.

PREMENSTRUAL SYNDROME AND MENOPAUSE

Karen is a 29-year-old mother of two who suffers from severe PMS. In the ten days prior to her menstrual cycle, Karen becomes very irritable and "weepy. " During this time, she frequently gets headaches that put her in bed for the day. She craves sweets and hides bags of M&Ms around the house. Her husband complains that throughout this time she is short of temper with him and yells at the children. Karen knows the chocolate is responsible for a weight gain, but says she can't stop the snacking. She asks her gynecol ogist for advice.

PMS affects teenagers as well as their menopausal mothers and embraces all social classes and ethnic groups. The disease has far reaching impact, since it is not only the woman with PMS who suffers, but it is often a great ordeal for her partner, family, friends, and workmates.

Premenstrual syndrome, otherwise not so lovingly called PMS, consists of varying symptoms that commence a few days before menstruation and completely pass after menstruation has ended. Furthermore, in order to fully qualify as PMS, the symptoms must not start more than 14 days prior to the onset of menstruation and must increase in intensity so that the worst distress is felt immediately before the heaviest of the bleeding begins. The symptoms can be anticipated with cyclic regularity. The severity of PMS symptoms ranges from mild to incapacitating. Symptoms can occur for only one or two days or may begin at ovulation and continue until the onset of menstruation. Actually, dysmenorrhea (or menstrual cramps) is not considered a symptom of PMS. However, a woman can experience both PMS and dysmenorrhea.

The symptoms of PMS are numerous and varied. They can include premenstrual tension, often called PMT, which encompasses irritability, depression, anger, wide mood changes, temper tantrums, hostility, and crying spells. Physical symptoms can include headache, both tension and migraine types; asthma; epilepsy; joint pains; bloatedness; fluid retention; rhinitis; and acne and other complexion changes. Premenstrual syndrome may indeed be the world's most common disease, yet there is still no agreement among doctors as to its cause, whether it really *is* a disease, or, much less, the best way to treat its victims. Worldwide, there have been over 150 symptoms ascribed to PMS. No wonder there is such confusion, argument, and skepticism about the problem.

PMS affects teenagers as well as their menopausal mothers and embraces all social classes and ethnic groups. The disease has far-reaching impact, since it is not only the woman with PMS who suffers, but it is often a great ordeal for her partner, family, friends, and workmates. Nevertheless, there is good news along with the bad, in that a wide range of treatments exists to combat the multitude of symptoms afflicting PMS victims.

PMS appears to be a chronic condition that is most severe among women in their thirties. However, many women who are in their thirties when they obtain medical treatment for PMS report that their symptoms started years earlier and gradually worsened. This particular decade of the lifecycle is filled with stress for many women: raising children, holding a job, and maintaining a household. Perhaps these same years may be a time when stress-responsive hormones reach their peak sensitivity in women.

PMS and the Sugar Connection

In a diet study of 853 university students, researchers found that the prevalence and severity of PMS was associated with high intakes of sugar-containing foods and drinks. Large amounts of sugar increase the loss of magnesium in the urine, and since a high sugar diet is often lacking in sufficient magnesium to begin with, this can lead to a mild magnesium deficiency. This magnesium deficiency may cause some of the symptoms of PMS, including the emotional symptoms, anxiety, insomnia, and depression, by decreasing levels of the neurotransmitter dopamine. The insulin response to a high-sugar diet can also lead to the suppression of ketoacids, compounds that help to clear excess sodium and water from the kidneys. This can result in water retention, which causes bloating, weight gain, breast tenderness, and edema in the face and extremities.

Serotonin and Pain

When Serotonin levels in the brain are low, the sensitivity to pain increases. This has been presented by some researchers as one contributing factor in premenstrual syndrome. The pain and irritability are perhaps related to a hormone-induced decrease in "Serotonergic" activity.

PMS and Serotonin

Is carbohydrate craving during the premenstrual phase another instance of self-medication? Of all the neurotransmitters studied to date, Serotonin appears to be the most important in the development of PMS. Indeed, PMS shares many of the features of other mood and anxiety disorders.

In an effort to clarify the role of Serotonin in PMS, 16 women were given both a tryptophan-free mixture (to cause low tryptophan levels or tryptophan depletion) and a placebo mixture during their follicular and luteal phases of two menstrual cycles. This tryptophan depletion aggravated the pre menstrual symptoms, particularly irritability, in one-half of the women with PMS. The authors also concluded that low levels of Serotonin may provoke symptoms in susceptible women, regardless of cycle phase. This study supports other research that has found Serotonin deficiency in premenstrual syndrome.

If low serotonin levels can cause PMS, what is the effect of Serotonin-increasing agents? As you might expect, the use of SSRis is not uncommon in treating women with PMS. The Serotonin reuptake inhibitors include fluoxetine (Prozac), sertraline (Zoloft), and paroxetine (Paxil). One study found that fluoxetine at a dose of 20 to 60 mg day was significantly superior to the placebo in reducing symptoms of tension, irritability, and dysphoria in women with PMS.

PMS and 5-HTP

As we have seen, treatment with the Serotonin reuptake inhibitors can cause many side effects. In one study of 64 women who were treated with fluoxetine for PMS, 17% reported sexual dysfunction. It's no wonder women are seeking an alternative treatment.

Supplemental 5-HTP is recommended for PMS by a wide variety of practitioners, including nutritionists, holistic physicians, psychiatrists, and naturopaths. Experience has taught them that it works best on the symptoms of anxiety, irritability, and depression. Take Karen, the woman at the beginning of the chapter. Her gynecologist was able to greatly reduce her symptoms by recommending 5-HTP and some dietary changes.

How much 5-HTP should be used for PMS? Dr. Christian Renna is a medical doctor who uses 5-HTP in his private practice for the treatment of PMS. He gave us this example.

I treated a 28-year-old mother of one who had significant irritability 7 to 10 days prior to her menstrual cycle and who refused to take prescription medication. She was treated with 5-HTP-a standing dose of 30 mg twice a day, with "as needed" doses of 15-20 mg throughout the days of her PMS. That made a total of 50-70 mg day. She was able to control her irritability and emotionalism during her menstrual phase without the use of prescription medications.

Dr. Elisa Lotter is a naturopath who practices in Santa Barbara, California. She also uses 5-HTP with her patients.

"I use it for depression, anxiety, and sometimes pain. Because pain is something that if you increase the Serotonin level, pain is greatly reduced." She uses 5-HTP in conjunction with the natural hormone progesterone. "In the perimenopause, where the state is estrogen dominance, very often people will go into an eating disorder and I have found 5-HTP to be very useful in these cases."

Is carbohydrate craving during the pre menstrual phase another instance of self-medication? Of all the neurotransmitters studied to date, Serotonin appears to be the most important in the development of PMS. Indeed, PMS shares many of the features of other mood and anxiety disorders.

Today's women are under an immense pressure to be slim, even more so than in the past. It is no longer merely a popular trend to be cute and slim; it is now good business to be bright, attractive, and slim. Even though good looks and a muscular physique don't hurt men in the business world, they are not under the same degree of pressure to keep slim and trim. Women push themselves to the point of being malnourished in order to stay several sizes too small.

Low-calorie diets can lead to tryptophan depletion. This can be the result of too low a protein intake. Jennifer is an example of this.

Jennifer was a petite, active woman only 5 feet 1 inch tall. In order to keep her slim figure, Jennifer stopped eating meat, dairy, and fish, limited herself to 800-1,000 calories a day, and exercised at the gym faithfully. Although she looked healthy, a diet analysis indicated that Jennifer was not eating enough protein. When her protein intake was increased, Jennifer's PMS symptoms were greatly relieved.

Sometimes Serotonin levels are the result of too low an intake of carbohydrates. This was the case with Denise.

Denise was a successful 40-year-old executive. Denise had read a popular diet book that said carbohydrates were bad for you. She believed that a high-protein diet would increase her tryptophan levels and decrease the terrible anxiety and depression that preceded her menstrual periods. She carefully constructed each meal and snack to be high in protein. However, instead of making things better, Denise found that the high protein diet exacerbated her symptoms.

At first glance, Denise seems to be on the right track. Many people who follow the high-protein diets that are now the fad believe they are increasing their tryptophan levels. However, the opposite is true. Denise has in fact lowered her tryptophan levels even more. Unlike Jennifer, who ate too little protein, Denise did not lack the raw materials for Serotonin; she lacked the ability to get the raw materials into her brain cells. Carbohydrates in the diet increase brain tryptophan levels by decreasing the competition for absorption from the other amino acids. A high-protein diet just increases the competition for tryptophan. The result is that there is an abundance of tryptophan and other amino acids in the blood, but not enough in the brain.

On the advice of her doctor, Denise ate a high-carbohydrate meal in the evening. She made sure that she ate only complex carbohydrates, along with some fat, to help reduce the large fluctuations in her insulin level. Denise also started to take 50 mg of 5-HTP before bed. After one week she increased this dose to 100 mg. Denise was delighted with the result. Not only did her cravings and irritability disappear, Denise found that she was now sleeping better.

Denise learned the hard way that no one macronutrient is "bad." Carbohydrates are just as important to the body as protein.

The Nay-Sayers

Of course, there are still a number of persons, both medical professionals as well as laypeople, who continue to believe that PMS is just an "all in the mind" phenomenon. Nowadays, most doctors and medical scientists accept that PMS exists as a disease process, although there is still much disagreement about its causes and methods of treatment. Sadly, though, a few doctors still tell PMS sufferers, 'Just pull yourself together, it isn't that bad!" Obviously, those are not doctors who have had PMS. Other doctors treat their PMS patients for simple depression or consider them "crocks." Still, most physicians today realize that PMS is real, a true cyclic illness brought about by actual cyclic, physical changes.

Nowadays, most doctors and medical scientists accept that PMS exists as a disease process, although there is still much disagreement about its causes and methods of treatment. Sadly, though, a few doctors still tell PMS sufferers, *"Just pull yourself together, it isn't that bad!" Obviously, those are not doctors who have had PMS.*

Ironically, many of the doubters are psychologists and psychiatrists who still tend to believe that all mood disorders are mainly caused by events in early life. It is hard to believe that any practicing psychiatrists refuse to accept the effectiveness of drugs in treating depression and schizophrenia; nevertheless, a die-hard few are still disinclined to accept the chemical concept of psychiatry. Since it is being proven more and more frequently that mental states and functions are governed by hormones, neurotransmitters, and other chemicals, this leaves less room for psychoanalysis as a viable treatment. It is difficult for some people to give up old habits!

Surprisingly, certain of the more extreme feminists also refuse to accept PMS as a disease entity. To them, the existence of PMS means that women are not the equals of men; they believe that this is a classification created by men and designed to help prove the inequality of the sexes. Fortunately, the extremists among the feminists and die-hard psychoanalysts are a small minority. Too many feminists have PMS and know damn well it isn't in their minds, and too many psychiatrists practice good medicine and know that body chemistry is not a figment of their imagination; it is, rather, a mediator of the functions of the mind.

Some estimates say that about 10% of menstruating women experience severe premenstrual symptoms. While PMS can occur at any point in a menstruating woman's lifetime, it generally appears in her late 20s and 30s.

How You Can Tell if You Experience PMS

At present, there is no medical or laboratory test that

definitely reveals the presence of PMS. It is essential to keep a daily calendar to record the symptoms you experience. If you find that symptoms recur about 7 to 14 days before your period and you have a symptom-free phase after menstruation, then you are probably experiencing PMS. Seek medical help for further evaluation and treatment if these symptoms are severe or debilitating.

More Women Now Suffer from PMS

It does indeed appear that there are a lot more PMS cases today than when I first began my medical practice over 45 years ago. Or did we just not talk about it as a disorder then? Was there actually less PMS, or did we just call it other things? We certainly didn't call it premenstrual syndrome, because that name wasn't around then. We didn't relate the symptoms to the monthly period; we just saw mood changes that came with the "curse." A lot of women were made to believe they just couldn't cope with all of the pressures of running a household. Naive, weren't we?

But, yes, I do think there is a lot more PMS today. Even though we didn't know how to diagnose it in my early days as a physician, I think there has been a steady increase in the disease since we started calling it PMS a couple of decades ago. Possibly, the numbers are increasing just because the problem is more openly discussed. This surely has something to do with it, but it is not the only reason for the rise in cases. I think there are several factors making the symptoms of PMS more intense and widespread, most of which are due to lifestyle changes among women today. Modern women are having fewer pregnancies and they are beginning to undergo those pregnancies at a much later age. They are exposed to more stress as they take on responsible and competitive positions in the workplace. In addition, the contraceptive pill has synthetically altered the normal hormonal cycling in the female body. Even diet may be contributing to the problem, as women join the fast-food, high-saturated-fat, eat-on-the-run world of business. Add to this the fact that more women are smoking today, and you have a formula for a health disaster.

We think there are several factors making the symptoms of PMS more intense and widespread, most of which are due to lifestyle changes among women today. Modern women are having fewer pregnancies and they are beginning to undergo those pregnancies at a much later age. They are exposed to more stress as they take on responsible and competitive positions in the workplace. In addition, the contraceptive pill has synthetically altered the normal hormonal cycling in the female body. Even diet may be contributing to the problem, as women join the fast-food, high-satu rated-fat, eat-on-the-run world of business. Add to this the fact that more women are smoking today, and you have a formula for a health disaster.

Before the advent of reliable and convenient forms of contraception, most women were pregnant for a large percentage of their fertile years. Not only were they pregnant more frequently, missing anywhere from zero to 45 or more of their periods between the ages of 18 to 35, they missed even more periods if they breast-fed their young. Today, a woman might have 12 periods a year up to the age of 30 before she even *thinks* of motherhood. A century ago, she might well have had 12 total periods in that same time span, due to multiple pregnancies and with prolonged breast feeding used as a means of contraception. She might have had only a tenth of the chances to feel PMS that the modern woman gets. Now, I'm not suggesting that you stay pregnant so that you miss out on the symptoms of PMS; I'm just suggesting that today's lifestyle lends itself to the diagnosis of more prevalent PMS. We would have seen more of it in the past if we'd given it a chance to show itself and had a single name for it.

PMS and Supplements

Many women have reported the successful reduction of PMS symptoms as a result of using nutritional supplements such as vitamins B6 and E, zinc, magnesium, and essential fatty acids; herbs such as chasteberry, and black cohosh. European women have used 5-HTP successfully to reduce some of the symptoms of PMS but not to cure the disorder. If you are interested in trying nutritional supplements, check with your health care professional or your pharmacist for the recommended dosages.

PMS and Exercise

Regular exercise can help to relieve the stress that comes with PMS. Regular aerobic exercise increases the body's supply of endorphins, nature's natural sedatives; improves circulation; and promotes cardiovascular health. Exercise also helps to release pent-up anxiety and tension and induce good quality sleep, which is essential during PMS. Supplements of 5-HTP also can help to induce and maintain a good night's rest.

Treatments for PMS

There is no one treatment for PMS because the symptoms are very individual and the exact cause of this condition is not known. Treatments that may help include vitamin supplements, dietary changes, and drug therapy. Learning to recognize the symptoms is an important step. Psychological counseling to increase a woman's coping skills, in conjunction with medical treatment, may help. PMS support groups can be extremely beneficial.

Dealing with stress more effectively through techniques such as meditation, yoga, and deep muscle relaxation may reduce PMS discomfort. Less formal methods such as sitting in a quiet room, listening to relaxing music, talking with a friend, or even a leisurely hot bubble bath may take the edge off symptoms. Learning how to cope with stressful situations can be helpful. Some women suffering from PMS have found that taking "time out," or a brief break from an argument, makes it possible to handle the problem instead of getting out of control and making it worse. Learning to anticipate the worst premenstrual days and not schedule stressful activities on those days is another stress-reducing approach that works for some women.

Many of the symptoms of PMS are mediated by Serotonin and if it is deficient, taking supplements of 5-HTP may help to replenish it so that the symptoms can be reduced.

Menopause

Menopause finally brings an end to premenstrual symptoms. This remedy may be either natural menopause or a surgical menopause, with removal of the ovaries. There is some evidence that PMS symptoms gradually decrease from their peak levels of severity even before menopause.

During menopause, the Serotonin levels change. Whether the body is being affected by the hormones progesterone or estrogen, we're not quite sure. Menopause brings its own list of symptoms.

Menopause and Serotonin

Angela is 52 years old and has come to her doctor complaining of hot flashes, dryness in her vaginal tissues, and emotional symptoms. Her first concern is the vaginal dryness because this has led to a decrease in sexual activity between her and her husband. The emotional problems are running a close second. "One minute I'm fine, the next I'm all upset and crying. The smallest problem seems to set me off on a crying spree." Angela s husband is at a loss to know what to do. "Every time I try to help, it only makes her more angry. I'm in trouble when I try to help and in trouble if I ignore the problem. I can't win." Since menopause can cause symptoms of a Serotonin dysfunction, Angela's physician gave her a prescription for Prozac a Serotonin reuptake inhibitor.

Angela has two sets of symptoms here. The physical symptoms of vaginal dryness and hot flashes are probably due to a hormone imbalance. The emotional symptoms of anxiety and depression may be the result of a Serotonin dysfunction and therefore amenable to treatment with 5-HTP.

5-HTP and Menopause

We asked Dr. Renna for his opinion on the use of 5-HTP for menopause:

"Perimenopause and menopause are filled with a constellation of biochemical changes. You cannot realistically expect that one supplement such as 5-HTP or one neurochemical such as Serotonin could resolve all symptoms. But you would expect that some symptoms would be improved, and, in fact, these symptoms of irritability and depression have been improved in women- I have treated for menopausal and premenopausal discomfort."

In his practice he has found that 5-HTP works well to reduce the symptoms of anxiety that often accompany menopause.

Let's return to the case of Angela.

After six months on Prozac Angela reported that her mood swings had disappeared. Unfortunately so did her sex drive. She went to see a naturopathic physician to find an alternative. Her new doctor recommended that she tapered her off of the Prozac and substitute 5-HTP. After three months on 5-HTP, she reports that her mood swings have evened out and her sex drive has returned.

Dr. Elisa Lotter talks about the anxiety some women experience as they approach menopause. "People really want to self-medicate themselves. People are saying, 'Look, I'm much more anxious.' They are very fearful about menopause, both from a physiological level and a psychological level, particularly where I practice, a very affluent area where we have a lot of film industry people. We have the most beautiful women in the world, and the biggest fear is, I'm getting old, I'm feeling old, I'm looking old, I will not get a part, and so on. I think 5-HTP can be very valuable in this sense because it ameliorates a lot of that anxiety about getting old."

While the answer to many of the physical symptoms of menopause are beyond the scope of this book, the mental problems can very well be treated by supplements of 5-HTP alone.

More From Othniel

<u>Health</u>

5 HTP The Serotonin Connection:
*The Natural Supplement that helps
you be in control of your mind and body!*
ISBN: 1519148445
5-HTP and Depression Management:
Available in Kindle Only
5HTP and Memory Loss Management with:
Available in Kindle Only
5 HTP PMS and Menopause:
Available in Kindle Only
Coping with Arthritis:
ISBN: 151941353X
Coping with BPH:
*Benign Prostatic Hypertrophy
Male, over 45, you probably have it!*
Available in Kindle Only
Coping with Colorectal Cancer:
*Prevention and Cure of theSecond Leading
Cause of Cancer Deaths*
Available in Kindle Only
Coping with Fibromyalgia:
It's not in your head, it's a disease!
ISBN: 1519438311

Coping with Prostate Cancer:
Prevention and Cure
of Man's Most Common Cancer
ISBN: 1519438737

Heart of a Woman:
Prevetion and Cure of the #1 Killer in Women
ISBN: 1519441533

Heavy and Healthy:
Forget Your Weight and Get Fit!
ISBN: 1519495412

Quit Smoking Now!:
The Program to Help You
Quit Smoking Now and Forever!
ISBN: 1519495781

Sharpening the Aging Mind:
Methods, Tricks & Tips to
Keep Your Mind Super Sharp
ISBN: 1519496028

Sleep Disorders Management:
Available in Kindle Only

The Second half begins at 50:
Your Longevity Handbook
ISBN: 1519496389

Walk!:
Walk Your Way to Great Health & Long Life
Available in Kindle Only

Weight & Appetite Management:
Available in Kindle Only

Relationships:

Adultery Case Histories:
Why People Cheat on Their Partners
Available in Kindle Only

Communing with the Dead:
Death Needn't Part You
ISBN: 1519190085

Foreplay:
The True Focus of Great Sex
ISBN: 1519440979

Sex in the Golden Years:
The Best Sex Ever, Stay Sexually Active for Life
ISBN: 1519495927

The Big O:
Male & Female Multiple Orgasms
ISBN: 1519496109

The Hospice Experience:
Making Your Most Important Final Decision
ISBN: 1519496281

When Your Spouse Dies:
A widow's & widower's handbook
ISBN: 151949646X

Jewish Fiction

Padre Pio:
The Capuchin – the life of Padre Pio -
St. Pio of Pietrelcina
Sex, Horror & Violence vs. Unyielding Faith!
ISBN: 1519495684

Seed of Avraham:
A 4000 Year History of the Jewish Family...
ISBN: 1519495811

Shtetl:
> *The Story of a Life No More...*
> *As told from the hereafter*
> **ISBN: 1519496036**

The Cartographer:
> *1492*
> **ISBN: 151949615X**

The Condemned Voyage:
> *The S.S. St. Louis - 1939*
> **Available in Kindle Only**

The Crusades:
> *The Jewish World of the 12th Century*
> **Available in Kindle Only**

The Death of Berlin:
> *A Story of Hollocaust Survival and Revenge*
> **Available in Kindle Only**

The Remnant:
> *The Jewish Resistance in WWII*
> **ISBN: 1519496346**

The Uprising of Babi Yar:
> *The Syrets Deathcamp*
> **Available in Kindle Only**

Miscellaneous

Guaranteed Routes to Success for Writers:
> *A Road Map Through Today's*
> *Dramatic Changes in Publishing*
> **Available in Kindle Only**

Joy of Volunteering:
> *Working and Surviving in Developing Countries*
> **ISBN: 1519495587**

So You Want to Write a Book:
> **ISBN: 1519496079**

If you liked this book,

please leave a reviwe for it on

Amazon.com

Thank you!!!

Also available in Kindle